INTERVENTION WITH HYPERACTIVE CHILDREN
A Case Study Approach

INTERVENTION WITH HYPERACTIVE CHILDREN
A Case Study Approach

Marvin J. Fine, Ph.D.
School Psychology Training Program
University of Kansas
Lawrence, Kansas

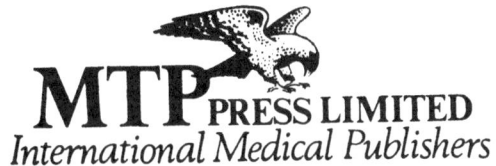

MTP PRESS LIMITED
International Medical Publishers

Published in the UK and Europe by
MTP Press Limited
Falcon House
Lancaster, England

Published in the US by
SPECTRUM PUBLICATIONS, INC.
175-20 Wexford Terrace
Jamaica, N.Y. 11432

ISBN-13: 978-94-011-6286-9   e-ISBN-13: 978-94-011-6284-5
DOI: 10.1007/978-94-011-6284-5

Acknowledgment

Appreciation is expressed to the many contributors to this book. They all share a genuine concern for the hyperactive child and are making their respective contributions to assisting this child and his family.

I have benefited from the stimulation and support of my colleagues. In particular, John Poggio and Neil Salkind, through their own research with hyperactivity, have demonstrated a high standard of scholarship. They have both been readily available to discuss issues and to share ideas.

Jacalyn Wright assisted me greatly in the editing of manuscripts, as did Penni Holt and Roger Maitland. Peggy Miller and Gayle Robb were kind and patient with me as they typed and retyped the manuscript.

The result of the efforts and contributions of these individuals is a book that should be of great value to persons working with hyperactive children.

M. J. F.

Contributors

JOAN E. BACKMAN
Department of Psychology
Carleton University
Ottawa, Ontario

JOY PATRICIA BURKE, Ed.D.
Human Development and Psychological
   Services
University of North Carolina—
   Chapel Hill
Chapel Hill, North Carolina

STEPHEN T. DeMERS, Ed.D.
School Psychology Program
University of Kentucky
Lexington, Kentucky

NORMA ESTRADA, Ph.D.
Psychology Department
Everett Gladman Hospital
Oakland, California

H. BRUCE FERGUSON, Ph.D.
Department of Psychology
Carleton University
Ottawa, Ontario

A. J. FINCH, Ph.D.
Department of Psychology
Virginia Treatment Center for Children
Medical College of Virginia
Virginia Commonwealth University
Richmond, Virginia

MARVIN J. FINE, Ph.D.
Department of Educational
   Psychology and Research
University of Kansas
Lawrence, Kansas

LINDA HALL JACKSON, M.D.
Child Psychiatry
The Menninger Foundation
Topeka, Kansas

PHILIP C. KENDALL, Ph.D.
Department of Psychology
University of Minnesota
Minneapolis, Minnesota

KATHERINE GLENN KENT, M.S.
Family Therapy Training Program
The Menninger Foundation
Topeka, Kansas

MIMI LUPIN, M.A.
Self Management Tapes
Houston, Texas

JEAN MAYO, M.S.
Feingold Association of the U.S.A.
Houston, Texas

CHRISTOPHER R. MILAR, Ph.D.
Division for Disorders of Development
    and Learning
University of North Carolina—
    Chapel Hill
Chapel Hill, North Carolina

MARY MIRA, Ph.D.
Children's Rehabilitation Unit
University of Kansas Medical Center
Kansas City, Kansas

EUNICE NELSON, M.Ed.
Department of Educational Psychology
Wichita State University
Wichita, Kansas

A. LEE PARKS, Ph.D.
Department of Special Education
University of Idaho
Moscow, Idaho

NANCY L. PETERSON, Ph.D.
Department of Special Education
University of Kansas
Lawrence, Kansas

JOHN P. POGGIO, Ph.D.
Department of Educational
    Psychology and Research
University of Kansas
Lawrence, Kansas

JEAN L. PYFER, P.E.D.
Department of Health, Physical
    Education and Recreation
University of Kansas
Lawrence, Kansas

HERBERT J. RIETH, Ed.D.
Department of Special Education
Indiana State University
Bloomington, Indiana

NEIL J. SALKIND, Ph.D.
Department of Educational
    Psychology and Research
University of Kansas
Lawrence, Kansas

R. L. SHERBENOU, Ph.D.
Department of Special Education
Purdue University
Lafayette, Indiana

BARBARA J. THOMPSON, M.A.
Department of Education
Baker University
Baldwin, Kansas

RONALD TRITES, Ph.D.
Department of Psychiatry and Psychology
University of Ottawa
Neuropsychology Laboratory
Royal Ottawa Hospital
Ottawa, Ontario

HELEN TRYPHONUS, M.Sc.
Department of Health and Welfare
Health Protection Branch
Ottawa, Ontario

FRED H. WALLBROWN, Ph.D.
Department of Counseling and
    Personnel Services
Kent State University
Kent, Ohio

VIVIEN J. WORSTER, M.A.
Indiana Department of Public
    Instruction
Division of Innovative Education
Indianapolis, Indiana

Preface

Hyperactivity has historically been a major concern of parents and teachers. Over the years, the term has come to mean many things to different persons. For some, the term is synonymous with "brain damage," and the prescribed course of treatment is medical. For others, the term is a catch-all, covering almost any behaviors that are found to be obtrusive or disruptive by the child's caretakers. In recent years, there has been a great outcry by some over the use and abuse of the term as a justification for controlling the child. Others have expressed great concern over the excessive, inappropriate, or poorly monitored use of drug therapy with regard to hyperactivity.

The current interest in hyperactive children is reflected in several major books (Cantwell, 1975; Feingold, 1975; Fine, 1977; Ross and Ross, 1976; Wender, 1973; Safer and Allen, 1976; Stewart and Olds, 1973). The number of published papers and symposia over the last several years is also voluminous.

The main questions posed by practitioners revolve around intervention with the hyperactive child. The growing literature on intervention has identified a variety of approaches with demonstrated utility; including drug therapy, behavior modification, biofeedback, sensory-motor training, cognitive training, environmental manipulations, and family therapy.

The major text sources cited include recommendations and descriptions of intervention approaches with the hyperactive child. But most fall short of extensive case-study material that details the thinking behind the intervention and the specific steps that were actually followed. For the school psychologist, counselor, learning consultant, and teacher looking for specific direction, there is a void of good resources. Blanco's text on program prescriptions (Blanco, 1972) is a model of one kind of a "how-to-do-it" approach; while this approach has demonstrable value, the reader is required to have an already functional frame of reference into which specific and unelaborated suggestions can fit. In contrast, the booklet by Conner (1974) presents an extensive detailing of classroom procedures; the activities discussed, however, seem to be more of a novel, attention-getting nature to be used with an entire class of students, rather than specific children whose hyperactivity may interfere with extensive and cooperative group involvement.

This book of case studies is intended to meet the needs of persons working with hyperactive children who are interested in learning about specific intervention approaches. The book should serve as a source book of concepts and procedures on intervention, with enough detailing of rationale and intervention to expand the practitioner's repertoire of strategies for intervention. It emphasizes intervention in educational as well as home settings, and as such, places emphasis on the kinds of interventions that non-medical persons can affect. The book should also be of great value to physicians who may be seeking alternatives or supplements to a pharmaceutical approach. Accordingly, drug studies per se were omitted, although drug treatment is discussed.

The orientation of the chapters is first to present an initial introduction to literature on hyperactivity; touching on the historical issues, treatment efficacy studies, and the current scene; with regard to concepts of etiology, developmental course, and intervention. This is followed by several chapters concerned with specific intervention themes. For example, there are chapters that give detailed case studies on intervention via behavioral strategies, sensory-motor training, biofeedback and relaxation procedures, psychotherapeutic approaches, and classroom curriculum modifications. The usefulness of the book as a sourcebook is enhanced by the organization of the case studies. Each case study is presented in the following framework: 1. Current Problem, 2. Background Information, 3. Intervention, and 4. Conclusions. This framework should provide the reader with ample information to correlate the case study child with the children he is concerned about. Each chapter has an orienting introduction, with key references cited.

The measurement of hyperactivity is important if we are to determine whether changes have occurred as a result of an intervention. The chapter by Salkind and Poggio represents a compendium and critical analysis of instruments for assessing hyperactivity. The last chapter of the book summarizes some important considerations in diagnosis and intervention; the need to view the child holistically, the importance of a comprehensive and differential diagnosis, and collaborative planning by the involved persons are stressed.

References

BLANCO, R. F. *Prescriptions for Children with Learning and Adjustment Problems.* Springfield, Ill.: Charles C Thomas, 1972.

CANTWELL, D. P. (Ed.) *The Hyperactive Child.* New York: Spectrum Publications, 1975.

CONNER, J. P. *Classroom Activities for Helping Hyperactive Children.* New York: Center For Applied Research in Education, 1974.

FINE, M. J. (Ed.) *Principles and Techniques of Intervention with Hyperactive Children.* Springfield, Ill.: Charles C Thomas, 1977.

FEINGOLD, B. F. *Why Your Child is Hyperactive.* New York: Random-House, 1975.

ROSS, D. M. and ROSS, S. A. *Hyperactivity: Research, Theory, and Action.* New York: John Wiley, 1976.

SAFER, D. J. and ALLEN, R. P. *Hyperactive Children: Diagnosis and Management.* Baltimore, Md.: University Park Press, 1975.

SCHRAG, P. and DIVOKY, D. *The Myth of the Hyperactive Child.* New York: Pantheon Books, 1975.

STEWART, M. A. and OLDS, S. W. *Raising a Hyperactive Child.* New York: Harper & Row, 1973.

WENDER, P. W. *The Hyperactive Child: A Handbook for Parents.* New York: Crown Publishers, 1973.

Contents

Part III   *Measurement, Diagnosis, and Intervention*

Part I
INTRODUCTION

CHAPTER 1

The Hyperactive Child

The hyperactive child is surely unique in the extent to which he has become a source of concern for parents and professionals. The last decade, in particular, has witnessed an acceleration of books, articles, and proposals of treatments for this child. Materials advocating particular viewpoints on cause and treatment of hyperactivity are readily available, although, quite clearly, there has not yet been a definitive and final statement on the subject.

The popularity of the term, its related myths, and the lack of closure on questions of etiology and efficacious intervention, are reminiscent of Louis Carroll's description of the hunt for "snarks" and the eventual discovery of a "boojum". Both "snarks" and "boojums," of course, being mythical creatures, while the hyperactive child, many would argue, is real. Among persons working with these children, there seems to be a fairly narrow band of concerns: (a) The hyperactive child is both a problem to himself and others, and (b) There is a need to identify helpful ways of intervening. As already stated, greater divergence exists regarding questions of cause and efficacious intervention.

Cruikshank's comments of a decade ago are still relevant today. "Hyperactive children by reason of their concomitant learning and management problems constitute one of the most perplexing issues to teachers and administrators and indeed to emotionally normal children within the school" (Cruikshank, 1967, p. 48). Home and family relationships are equally problematic. Wender (1973) and Stewart and Olds (1973) have spoken at length about the frustrations of parents. It is not unusual to find parents of children who have been hyperactive since early childhood feeling virtually helpless in managing the child's behavior.

The magnitude of the problem is reflected by estimates of over one million hyperactive children in the public schools (Eisenberg, 1973). Because of problems of definition, it is virtually impossible to obtain an accurate figure. But in reviewing teacher descriptions of handicapped children (Keogh, Tchir, and Windeguth-Behn, 1974), behavior patterns of learning disabled children (Paraskevopoulos and McCarthy, 1970), and the common symptoms of children referred to mental health clinics (Rogers, Lilienfeld, and Pasamanick, 1955), the term "hyperactive" recurs at a high frequency.

An extremely thorough and systematic attempt to ascertain the prevalence of hyperactivity was reported by Lambert, Sandoval and Sassone (1978). These authors considered both different definitions of hyperactivity and the reports from different sources; namely the home, the school, and physicians. They arrived at a maximum prevalence rate of 12 to 13 percent of the school population as being defined by at least one of the sources. Interestingly, when all three sources were considered as a single definition, the incidence of hyperactivity dropped drastically to just over 1 percent. This seems to speak to the differential behavior of children in different settings and the varying tolerance for the child's behavior by the caretaking persons. Low socioeconomic children were over-represented, while middle socioeconomic children were under-represented in the identified sample of hyperactive children. Boys were six to eight times more represented than girls.

Some additional interesting findings of this study were that (a) there are not more hyperactive children today that in the past, (b) prevalence does not seem to increase with age, and (c) the diagnosis of hyperactivity does not necessarily follow the child through his elementary school experiences.

The frequency of the diagnosis of hyperactivity accelerates once the child enters the public schools, and this would seem related to the child being "out of synch" with the demands of the school setting. "Sit still; be quiet; pay attention" are statements that characterize most educational settings. Our society puts a positive value on children who are able to attend, complete tasks, and learn. Even so-called "open" classrooms are not permissive settings where children are permitted to follow their own impulses. There is still a structure to the environment with implicit and explicit expectations regarding student behavior. Children who are relatively immobile and withdrawn may also exhibit learning and mental health problems, but in some ways they are more tolerable to parents and educators than children "on the go" or children who fidget, have difficulty attending, and who may chronically disrupt others.

In coping with hyperactive children, the aspect of control for control's sake is present. Schrag and Divoky (1973, p. xii) claimed that there are over one million children on medication, presumably with the main objective of making them more manageable. Hyperactivity in children is of grave concern to parents, teachers, and physicians. It also surfaces many ethical and social problems associated with the implications of labeling and with the basis on which we decide to manage children's behaviors. Recent articles (Cole and Moore, 1976; Schnackenberg, 1977) have called for a reassessment of the "condition" and the more judicious use of intervention strategies.

A Historical Perspective on the Concept of Hyperactivity

It is possible to reach far back, even in folklore, to find references to excessively active children. But for the professional community, it appears to have been the observation of a relationship between excessive physical activity and neurological conditions that heralded a "conceptual view of the condition" (Ebaugh, 1923; Kahn and Cohen, 1934). The creation of a syndrome, or definable "medical" condition, as opposed to viewing hyperactivity solely as a symptom, generated an outpouring of literature on etiology and management.

A cursory review of the literature will quickly reveal that the term "hyperactivity" is defined and used differently by various practitioners and researchers. It has even today achieved common usage with children who refer to a classmate as being "hyper".

Delong (1972) counted 37 different terms in use; including hyperactivity, hyperkinesis, hyperkinetic impulse disorder, and minimal brain dysfunction. While different terms are used, there does seem to be reasonably good agreement on a behavioral-descriptive level. A survey of teachers, psychologists, psychiatrists, social workers, and pediatricians sought to establish the extent of agreement on the behavioral characteristics of hyperactivity:

> Seventy-five percent or more of all groups felt the following six behaviors to be primary: fidgets and restless, inattentive, hard to manage, can't sit still, easily distracted, and low frustration. Medical professionals were concerned also with irritability, undisciplined, clumsy, poor sleeper, seems slow and awkward. (Schrager, Lindy, Harrison, McDermott and Killins, 1966, p. 636)

It is also interesting to note that even though the term "hyperactivity" and its common synonyms connote the child as being in constant movement, research has failed to support this notion (Pope, 1970). Safer and Allen (1976) point out that it is the hyperactive child's inability to sit quietly and pay attention when the activity requires it that becomes problematic. They concluded . . . "a better way of viewing the activity problem these children have is to state that they have difficulty modulating their activity level, particularly when they are expected to perform an abstract academic task" (p. 6).

Another consistently found aspect of hyperactivity is that boys predominate over girls, several to one (Stewart and Olds, 1973, p. 19; Lambert et al., 1978, p. 459). Lower IQ's are reported for hyperactive children as a group (Minde et al., 1971) but how the hyperactive behavior may have interfered with test performance is questionable. Also, while certain behavioral manifestations of the condition decrease with adolescence, there are often remaining problems of school learning and social adjustment (Minde et al., 1971).

A recent report of a ten-year follow-up study shed additional light on the developmental course of the hyperactive chlid (Weiss et al., 1978). Given the existing data on the problems these children experienced in adolescence, a variety of problems when they become young adults could be predicted. The Weiss et al. study (1978) confirmed these predictions in some respects, but also produced some surprising findings. The hyperactive subjects rated themselves lower than did the normal comparison group in several personal-social functioning areas. Additional negative findings were that the "hyperactive subjects had more car accidents . . . moved more frequently, and had a higher incidence of impulsive or immature personality traits. However, only a small minority had become chronic offenders of the law or seriously emotionally disturbed" (Weiss et al., p. 444).

In the important area of employment, the study revealed that employers viewed the hyperactive subjects to be as competent in the work setting as the normal matched control subjects. Not surprisingly, the teachers who had these children in their last year of high school rated them lower than the normals on items involving completing assignments, working independently, and relating to peers.

In relation to school learning problems among hyperactive children, Douglas (1972) reported a high incidence of failing grades by the time they were 12 years old. The exact nature of learning problems seems to vary among hyperactive children, but some explanatory hypotheses have been presented.

Attentional deficits have been identified by several researchers (Keogh, 1971; Alabiso, 1972; Douglas, 1972). Support for this hypothesis comes from research showing that under conditions of continuous reinforcement, hyperactive children perform as well as normals on a concept-learning task (Freibergs and Douglas, 1969), while under conditions of partial reinforcement, the quality of performance decreases. Keogh (1971) also described how the child's impulsiveness can lead to faulty decision-making which, in turn, can affect learning. The writings of Kagan on cognitive tempo (Kagan, 1965) are cited as evidence for this hypothesis.

The possibility of neurological impairment affecting learning is also cited by Keogh, but rejected. She is willing to attribute some of the child's behavior problems to organic causes, but was unable to find evidence to support an organic basis to learning problems.

Hyperactivity, as defined by its symptoms, can vary in intensity and in its effects on the child. Not every hyperactive child may need a special program. The demands of the environment certainly have a lot to do with how severe the symptoms are viewed. In a permissive family or classroom, children who are mildly or moderately hyperactive by someone's definition may be viewed simply as energetic children who like to shift through different tasks and activities. In another classroom, the same observations would produce a different set of conclusions; such as, "he never finishes tasks and his attention constantly wanders." On a positive note, Stewart and Olds (1973) describe the childhood of several highly successful individuals. By applying some usual definitions and criteria, such "greats" as Thomas Edison, Huey Long, Sergei Rachmaninoff, and many others would have been considered hyperactive.

Causes of Hyperactivity

A review of the literature identifies three main themes regarding the cause of hyperactivity: organic, psychological, and developmental. The ensuing discussion will overview the evidence and issues associated with each position.

The Organic Position

The observed link between encephalitis and hyperactivity encouraged an "organic" view of the condition, which in turn argued for medical treatment (i.e., medication). Even the educational programing proposed by Strauss and Lehtinen (1948) that involved destimulating the learning environment was based on beliefs about brain functioning.

A continuing problem for the proponents of a "brain damage" or "brain malfunctioning" hypothesis, is the lack of adequate and direct supportive evidence. For example, one study considered 100 children referred to a clinic with hyperactivity as one of the complaints (Kenny et al., 1971). Neurological findings were considered normal in over half of the children. Forty-eight children evidenced "soft" neurological signs. The authors reported that a significant relationship was not obtained among the neurological examination, electroencephalographic findings, and final diagnosis.

Despite such findings as the Kenny et al. study, a number of experts have maintained an organic view of the condition (Cruikshank, 1967; Solomons, 1971). Safer and Allen (1976) reviewed a potpourri of historical and developmental features that distinguish between hyperactive and non-hyperactive children. A number of these features potentially relate causally or are associated otherwise with organic problems. These include a higher rate of prematurity, more frequent respiratory disorders after delivery, and more vaginal bleeding and preclampsia for mothers of hyperactives. Hyperactive children also experience more congenital disorders. In contrast to proponents of an "organic" position, Chess (1960) believed that only 15 percent of hyperactivity involved neurological factors, while Schmitt (1974) attributed only 1 percent of hyperactivity to organic factors.

Thomas et al. (1968) spoke to the relationship of hyperactivity and brain damage in a way that may add some light to the controversy.

The consequences of brain damage in childhood have tended to be discussed as though there regularly appears a single syndrome characterized by hyperkinesis, distractibility, perseveration, perceptual disturbance, emotional lability, atypical cognitive functioning, and disturbances in impulse control . . . the hyperkinetic syndrome does occur in some children as a direct consequence of central nervous system damage. At the same time, the behavioral sequelae of brain damage in childhood can be most diverse . . . no pattern of behavioral dysfunction can be considered to fit all brain-damaged children. (Thomas, Chess, and Birch, p. 135)

The Developmental Position

A prevailing view with a great deal of support is that hyperactivity is a developmental pattern emerging from an inborn temperament and predisposition to the condition (Werry, 1968; Safer and Allen, 1976; Wender, 1973; Thomas et al., 1968; and Schmitt et al., 1973). Anyone spending a short time observing newborns will witness a dramatic demonstration of the normal variance of infant behavior.

Thomas et al. (1968) has documented temperament differences in nine areas; activity level, rhythmicity, approach or withdrawal, adaptability, intensity of reaction, threshold of responsiveness, quality of mood, distractibility, and attention span to persistence. Clearly, if certain combinations of these temperament characteristics dominate, the child is likely to be considered difficult to manage.

Kagan's work on cognitive tempo (1965) underscored the difference in children on the dimension of impulsivity-reflectivity. Many of the subsequent studies generated by Kagan concerned the modifiability of impulsive behavior and are germaine to work with hyperactive children (Kendall and Finch, 1978; Messer, 1976; Egeland, 1976; and Denney, 1972).

The following statement by Wender (1973) represents one of the strongest statements this writer has found asserting the developmental nature of hyperactivity.

> In virtually all instances hyperactivity is the result of an inborn temperamental difference in the child. How the child is treated and raised can affect the severity of his problem but it cannot cause the problem. Certain types of raising may make the problem worse, certain types of raising may make the problem better. No forms of raising can produce HA problems in a child who is not temperamentally predisposed to them. (Wender, p. 31)

Another facet of the "temperament" position is its genetic component. There are studies that reported hyperactive patterns in different generations of a family (Cantwell, 1972; Morrison and Stewart, 1971).

The Psychological Position

There are also proponents of a psychological position on hyperactivity. When the hyperactive child is viewed as agitated, disruptive, irritable, emotionally labile, and emotionally over-reactive, it is not unreasonable to consider the psychological origins of the condition. Marwitt and Stenner (1972) spoke of a "hyper-reactive" child in the sense of the child reacting to his fears and anxieties. Friedland and Shilkret (1973) described "defensive hyperactivity" as behavior children exhibited to maintain psychological distance from others and to avoid close relationships.

A group of teachers concerned with hyperactive children were asked to describe a hyperactive-like child and an average child in their classroom

(Fine, 1978). By contrast, the hyperactive children exhibited substantially more behavior calculated to rebuff and elicit angry reactions from others. These findings coincide with the Friedland and Shilkret (1973) observations.

An organic or developmental view of hyperactivity would likely see the condition present since early childhood. It is interesting to note that Kenny and his co-workers (Kenny et al., 1971) found that over half of their 100 children had an onset of hyperactivity at age five or older. Kenny and his co-workers also reported other data that would support the view of the hyperactive pattern of disturbed children.

> Sixty-four percent of the families had evidence of major environmental pathology. Nearly one third of the children (31) lived in one-parent families or did not live with either parent. Thirty-eight of the families were considered to be overtly unstable, including history of parental institutionalization for emotional disturbance, alcoholism, drug addiction, or criminal acts. Environmental deprivation was noted in 14 homes. (Kenny et al., p. 620)

While other supportive evidence and opinion is available on psychological factors affecting the development of a hyperactive pattern (Stewart, 1970; Wunderlich, 1973), there are many who argue against psychological factors as being primary causal agents (Wender, 1973; Safer and Allen, 1976). Few would disagree that the hyperactive child is not vulnerable to personal and social problems. The issue is whether the hyperactive pattern is initially generated by organic or developmental factors, or by psychological factors. In many cases, it may be difficult to establish a clear-cut etiology. The psychological problems that the child is experiencing certainly ought to be addressed as a part of the intervention, rather than the emphasis being solely on reducing the symptoms of hyperactivity.

Implications for the Practitioner

Given the set of possibilities for causal factors, where does this leave the practitioner? Certainly, knowledge on the cause of a condition can generate specific, related interventions. But such knowledge may be easier to hypothesize than to actually support with data. Of note is a study by Conners (1973) in which he presented data differentiating children with minimal brain dysfunction into six group profiles. Each of the groups differed on their pattern of IQ, achievement, role learning, attentiveness, and impulse control.

More recently, Loney et al. (1978) identified two main dimensions along which hyperkinetic children could vary: aggression and hyperactivity. These two dimensions permitted four subgroupings; low aggression-high hyperactivity, high aggression-low hyperactivity, high aggression-high hyperactivity, and low aggression-low hyperactivity. This study utilized only boys drawn from a population of children involved in an ongoing study of the hyperkinetic/minimal-brain-damage syndrome, as defined by the authors.

The findings of Conners and Loney et al. have implications regarding the tendency to view hyperactive chlidren as a homogeneous group. While sharing some common features which resulted in the label "hyperactive", these children are likely to break down into many subgroups. Hyperactive children will vary in attentional deficits, learning problems, sensory-motor development, extent of family pathology, intellectual capabilities, and general personality characteristics. So, to talk about "the hyperactive child" as if he were a clearly definable entity is spurious. Other than in obvious cases (which may not really be obvious to everyone involved), the search for etiology has not proven productive in terms of efficacious intervention. Cantwell's conclusion that "The term 'hyperactive child syndrome' should be used to denote a behavioral syndrome only, with no implications as to etiology" (Cantwell, 1975, p. 12) may seem too limiting to some. But, unless etiology can be clearly established, effective intervention may best be developed by considering the child in the situation, and each child considered individually.

Viewpoints on Intervention

The literature has proliferated with ideas on intervention. This section will concern itself mainly with three popular approaches: environmental modification, drug management, and behavior modification.

Environmental Modification

Perhaps the most publicized intervention in educational settings, prior to the escalation of drug usage, was environmental modification oriented around destimulating the environment (Strauss and Lehtinen, 1947; Strauss and Kephart, 1955; Cruikshank et al., 1961; Cruikshank, 1967). The premise was that due to brain damage, the hyperactive child could not adequately organize and process environmental stimuli. He would confuse foreground with background stimuli, become distracted by extraneous elements, and, accordingly, be unable to focus productively on what was necessary; for example, the teacher's lecture or words on a page.

The program that logically followed this premise emphasized (a) blocking out the extraneous stimuli and (b) accentuating the stimulus value of what the child was supposed to attend to. The use of cubicles and austere rooms proliferated for a period of time, until the efficacy of this approach failed to be adequately documented. As with many of the approaches touched on in the literature, environmental destimulation seemed to work with some children, in some settings, some of the time.

Variations of this approach still are popular in educational settings. If a child is distractible or distracts others, there is a certain logic to separating the child from others and from excessive stimulation for a part of the day or for certain learning tasks. Often this environmental destimulation approach is coupled with a broader psychoeducational approach. In addition to cubicles, partitions, or selective seating, the child may receive specialized instructional consideration. Examples of this would be shorter assignments with more immediate feedback, using curricular materials consistent with the child's preferred learning modality (such as a visually based reading program for a child with auditory processing difficulties), and remedial efforts focused on the child's specific learning deficits.

A recent provocative paper by Zentall (1977) documented the failure of the "destimulation model." He proposed increasing the stimulation value of the classroom, based on the thesis that the hyperactive child was actually understimulated and that through his activity pattern was seeking stimulation. Zentall offered several specific suggestions for teachers, including the use of colors and patterns, task novelty and difficulty, and use of movement in the classroom.

Drug Management

Simultaneous with the interest in environmental designs in education, interest was being shown by physicians in the use of stimulant medication (Bradley, 1937; Bradley and Bowen, 1940; Bender and Cottingham, 1942). Initially, it seemed illogical to administer a stimulant to what appeared to be an overly stimulated person. But what was observed was a seemingly "paradoxical effect." That is, while stimulant drugs would heighten the activity level of adults, they seemed to slow down the activity level of hyperactive children. Fish (1975) addressed herself to this issue, challenging the concept of "paradoxical effect."

Fish pointed out that the effect only appears paradoxical at the behavioral level. Many hyperactive children are "under-aroused" in terms of their central nervous system. As a function of the under-arousal the children cannot attend or focus adequately and seem distracted. When the central nervous system is energized by the stimulant medication, the child is able to attend, to focus, and consequently to decrease the pattern of hyperactive behavior. Zentall's earlier stated position would support Fish's explanation.

Despite the early clinical observations of the effects of stimulant drugs, their widespread use did not occur until the late fifties and into the sixties. At that time, a number of reports on the indiscriminant use of drugs to control children were widely publicized, with much public alarm. This led to a national conference sponsored by the Department of Health, Education, and Welfare (Freedman, 1971) to review the problem. The judicious use of stimulant medication with hyperactive children was supported, but there remained much public and professional concern over the use of medication (Sulzbacher, 1973; Delong, 1972). It was not surprising to see "high drama" invoked with such publicity attracting titles such as *"Drugging the American Child: We're Too Cavalier About Hyperactivity"* (Walker, 1974), *"Toward a Nation of Sedated Children"* (Divoky, 1973), *"A Slavish Reliance on Drugs: Are We Pushers For Our Own Children?"* (Offir, 1974), and finally, *"The Myth of the Hyperactive Child and Other Means of Child Control"* (Schrag and Divoky, 1975).

Beyond the contrived drama, there are a number of real problems and issues. What are the side effects of stimulant drugs? Do stimulant drugs encourage subsequent dependency on drugs by hyperactive children? How is self concept affected when a child believes he cannot control his own behavior but needs a drug? Do the drugs facilitate learning or are they mainly a behavioral control device?

An interesting study by Sprague and Sleator (1977) on the effects of medication on learning made the case for the necessity of a correct dosage. They found that .3 milligrams per kilogram of body weight enhanced learning, while a higher dosage decreased learning. However, there seems to be many more accounts of medication not appreciably affecting learning (Rie et al. 1976; Barkley and Cunningham, 1978; Gittelman-Klein and Klein, 1976). Barkley and Cunningham concluded from their review of the literature that when learning difficulties were the major complaint, medication was not likely to be useful. They believed that medication had its greatest usefulness when behavior management was the issue and the child's problematic behavior had resisted other interventions.

Behavior Modification

Systematic behavior modification has emerged as a popular alternative or supplementary treatment to drug management. Simmons (1975) presented three arguments for considering behavioral strategies. The first concerned the earlier stated questions regarding possible side effects of medication, especially on physical growth, and the encouragement of a drug-dependent pattern in the child. Simmons was also concerned that learning under drug state conditions may not transfer to when the child is in a non-drug state.

Simmons' second area of concern related to the need to see the hyperactive child as part of a family system and a broader social system. There is an interaction of the child with the larger system that includes perceptions and expectations. Therefore, the system, as well as the child alone, needs some attention and modification. Drugs alone would seem to establish the child as the sole "patient."

The third factor Simmons discussed was the differential responsiveness of hyperactive children to medication. For some children, the medication does not substantially affect the hyperkinesis. Also, for many hyperactive children, their problem areas extend beyond the classroom or specific home management situations to include, for example, peer relationships and following rules. So, just to reduce the hyperactive behavior will not necessarily improve these other problem areas. Therefore, some forms of behavior management seem necessary.

There are a wide variety of behavioral approaches with ample demonstration of their potential effectiveness (Safer and Allen, 1976; Reith, 1977; Allyon et al., 1975; Simmons, 1975). But behavioral procedures are not without their critics. Charges of "dehumanizing children," using a "mechanistic approach," and creating "automatons" who, like Pavlov's dog, will salivate on cue, have been levied. A main danger does seem to lie, as with medication, in the "control for control's sake" orientation to behavior modification. The insightful article by Winett and Winkler (1972) subtitled "be still, be quiet, be docile" captures the essence of this charge. However, there is growing evidence that the principles of behavior modification can be used effectively to design curricula and to help children achieve specific knowledge and skill competencies, as well as just managing excessive physical movements or "off task" behaviors.

Other Interventions

In addition to three most popular intervention strategies: environmental modification; stimulant drugs; and behavior management, a number of other potentially useful interventions have been described in the literature and most will be dealt with more extensively in subsequent sections of this book. Gaining rapidly in popularity through the fervor of parent groups is the diet management approach (Feingold, 1975). While there are some supportive data for the efficacy of the diet approach (Conners et al., 1976; Cook and Woodhill, 1976; Brenner, 1977), there are also some negative and mixed reports (Harley et al., 1978; Williams et al., 1978). Self-monitoring procedures involving systematic relaxation (Lupin et al., 1976; Putre et al., 1977; Klein, 1977) have demonstrated some effectiveness. Biofeedback is another promising area, but also one that has produced mixed results (Braud et al., 1975; Nall, 1973; Johnson, 1997). Based on beliefs about the perceptual-motor involvement of hyperactive children, various kinds of perceptual-motor training programs have been proposed. From the viewpoint of the hyperactive child experiencing attentional deficits, cognitive self-management procedures have been presented as potentially effective (Douglas, 1972; Douglas et al., 1976; Meichenbaum and Goodman, 1971). Other approaches of an individual and family psychotherapeutic nature will be discussed later in this book.

Summary

This chapter presented a historical perspective on hyperactivity. Some of the divergent opinions on etiology and intervention were discussed, along with the social and ethical issues raised by intervention. Definitional problems, incidence figures, and the developmental course of the hyperactive child were considered.

From this review a number of points can be distilled:

1. Hyperactivity in children often gets defined in relation to somconc's expectations.
2. There is an interaction between the child and his environment so as to diminish or accentuate the "annoyance" value of the child's symptoms.
3. Hyperactive children may share some common symptoms, but are likely to be quite different from each other in some important ways.
4. The potential causes of hyperactivity are varied and include organic, psychological, and constitutional factors.
5. The developmental course of hyperactivity is quite problematic for children and affects aspects of their personal and social adjustment through adolescence and at least into their young adult life.
6. A variety of interventions are available with medication, behavior modification and environmental planning being the major ones.
7. The data on efficacy of intervention is limited, considering the range of identified interventions.

8. Learning and perceptual motor problems often occur as a part of the hyperactivity syndrome.
9. Approximately 6 to 12 percent of school children could be classified as hyperactive, with boys predominating over girls.
10. Each hyperactive child needs to be considered and treated as an individual rather than serving as the target for generalizations about hyperactivity.
11. Professional assistance seems vital in order to plan interventions; support the child, his family, and teachers, and to evaluate the outcomes of intervention.

References

ALABISO, F. Inhibitory functions of attention in reducing hyperactive behavior. *Amer. J. Ment. Def.* 1972, 77:259-282.

ALLYON, T., LAYMAN, D., and KANDEL, H. J. A behavioral-educational alternative to drug control of hyperactive children. *J. Applied Behav. Anal.* 1975, 8:137-146.

BENDER, L., and COTTINGHAM, F. The use of amphetamine sulfate benzedrine in child psychiatry. *Amer. J. of Psychiat.* 1942, 99:116-121.

BARKLEY, R., and CUNNINGHAM, C. Do stimulant drugs improve academic performance of hyperkinetic children? *Clin. Pediatrics* 1978, 17:85-92.

BRADLEY, C. The behavior of children receiving benzedrine. *Amer. J. Psychiat.* 1937, 94:577-585.

BRADLEY, C., and BOWEN, M. School performance of children receiving amphetamine (benzedrine) sulfate. *Amer. J. Orthopsychiat.* 1940, 10:782-788.

BRAUD, L. W., LUPIN, M. N., and BRAUD, W. G. The use of electromyographic biofeedback in the control of hyperactivity. *J. Learning Dis.* 1975, 8:420-425.

BRENNER, A. A study of the efficacy of the Feingold diet on hyperkinetic children: Some favorable personal observations. *Clin. Pediatrics* 1977, 16:652-656.

CANTWELL, D. P. Epidemiology, clinical picture and classification of the hyperactive child syndrome. In Cantwell, D. P. (ed.), *The Hyperactive Child: Diagnosis, Management, Current Research.* New York: Spectrum Publications, 1975.

CANTWELL, D. P. Psychiatric illness in the families of hyperactive children. *Arch. Gen. Psychiat.* 1972, 27:414-417.

CHESS, S. Diagnosis and treatment of the hyperactive child. *N.Y.S. J. of Med.* 1960, 60:2379-2385.

COLE, S. D., and MOORE, S. F. The hyperkinetic child syndrome: The need for reassessment. *Child Psychiatry and Human Development* 1976, 7:103-112.

CONNERS, C. K. Psychological assessment of children with minimal brain dysfunction. *Annals of the N. Y. Acad. Sci.* 1973, 205:283-302.

CONNERS, C. K., GOYETTE, C., SOUTHWICK, D., LEES, J., and ANDROLUNIS, P. Food additives and hyperkinesis: A controlled doublebind experiment. *Pediatrics* 1976, 58:154-166.

COOK, P. S., and WOODHILL, J. The Feingold dietary treatment of the hyperkinetic syndrome. *Med. J. Australia* 1976, 2:85-90.

CRUICKSHANK, W. M. Hyperactive children: Their needs and curriculum. In Knoblock, P., and Johnson, J. L. (eds.), *The Teaching-Learning Process in Educating Emotionally Disturbed Children*. Syracuse: Syracuse University Press, 1967.

DELONG, A. R. What have we learned from psychoactive drug research on hyperactives? *Amer. J. Dis. in Child*. 1972, 123:105-119.

DENNEY, D. R. Modeling effects upon conceptual style and cognitive tempo. *Child Dev*. 1972, 43:105-119.

DIVOKY, D. Toward a nation of sedated children. *Learning*. 1973, 1:6-13.

DOUGLAS, V. Stop, look and listen: The problem of sustained attention and impulse control in hyperactive and normal children. *Canadian J. Behav. Sci*. 1972, 4: 259-282.

DOUGLAS, V. I., PARRY, P., MARTON, P., and GARSON, C. Assessment of a cognitive training program for hyperactive children. *J. Abn. Child Psychol*. 1976, 4:389-410.

EBAUGH, F. G. Neuropsychiatric sequelae of acute epidemic encephalitis in children. *Amer. J. Dis. in Child*. 1923, 25:89-97.

EGELAND, B. Training impulsive children in the use of more efficient scanning techniques. *Child Dev*. 1974, 45:165-171.

EISENBERG, L. The overactive child. *Hospital Practice*. 1973, 8:1-10.

FEINGOLD, B. F. *Why Your Child is Hyperactive*. New York: Random House, 1975.

FINE, M. J. Teacher ratings of the life positions of hyperactive children. Lawrence, Kan.: University of Kansas, 1978. Unpublished report.

FISH, B. Stimulant drug treatment of hyperactive children. In Cantwell, D. P. (ed.), *The Hyperactive Child: Diagnosis, Management, Current Research*. New York: Spectrum Publications, 1975.

FREEDMAN, D. Report on the conference on the use of stimulant drugs in the treatment of behaviorally disturbed young school children. Washington, D.C.: Department of Health, Education and Welfare.

FREIBERGS, V., and DOUGLAS, V. Concept learning in hyperactive and normal children. *J. Abn. Psychol*. 1969, 74:388-395.

FRIEDLAND, S. J., and SHILKRET, R. B. Alternative explanations of learning disabilities: Defensive hyperactivity. *Except. Child*. 1973, 40:213-215.

GITTELMAN-KLEIN, R., KLEIN, D. Methylphenidate effects in learning disabilities. *Arch. Gen. Psychiat*. 1976, 33:655-664.

HARLEY, J. P., RAY, R. S., TOMASI, L., EICHMAN, P. L., MATHEWS, C. G., CHUN, R., CLEELAND, C. S., and TRAISMAN, E. Hyperkinesis and food additives: testing the Feingold hypothesis. *Pediatrics*. 1978, 6:818-828.

JOHNSON, W. B. An experimental study of the effect of electromyography (EMG) biofeedback on hyperactivity in children. *Dissertation Abstracts*. 1977, 37: 4650-B.

KAGAN, J. Impulsive and reflective children: Significance of conceptual tempo. In Krumboltz, J. E. (Ed.), *Learning and the Educational Process*. Chicago: Rand McNally, 1965.

KAHN, E., and COHEN, L. H. Organic driveness—a brain stem syndrome and an experience—with case reports. *New England J. Med*. 1934, 210:748-756.

KENDALL, P. C., and FINCH, A. J. A cognitive-behavioral treatment for impulsivity: a group comparison study. *J. Cons. and Clin. Psychol*. 1978, 46:110-118.

KENNY, T. J., CLEMMENS, R. L., HUDSON, B. W., LENTZ, G. A., CICCI, R., and NAIR,

P. Characteristics of children referred because of hyperactivity. *J. Pediatrics.* 1971, 79:618-622.

KEOGH, B. Hyperactivity and learning disorders: review and speculation. *Except. Child.* 1971, 38:101-109.

KEOGH, B. K., TCHIR, C., and WINDEGUTH-BEHN, A. Teachers' perceptions of educationally high risk children. *J. Learning Dis.* 1974, 7:43-50.

KLEIN, S. A. Relaxation and exercise for hyperactive, impulsive children. *Dissertation Abstracts.* 1977, 37:6334.

LAMBERT, N. M., SANDOVAL, J., and SASSONE, D. Prevalence of hyperactivity in elementary school children as a function of social system definers. *Am. J. Orthopsychiat.* 1978, 48:446-463.

LONEY, J., LANGHORNE, J. E., PATERNITE, C. E. An empirical basis for subgrouping the hyperkinetic/minimal brain dysfunction syndrome. *J. Abn. Psychol.* 1978, 87:431-441.

LUPIN, M., BRAUD, L. W., BRAUD, W., and DUER, W. F. Children, parents and relaxation tapes. *Acad. Ther.* 1976, 12:105-113.

MARWITT, S. J. and STENNER, A. J. Hyperkinesis: delineation of two patterns. *Except. Child.* 1972, 38:401-406.

MEICHENBAUM, D. and GOODMAN, J. Training impulsive children to talk to themselves: A means of developing self control. *J. Abn. Psychol.* 1971, 77:115-126.

MESSER, S. B. Reflection—impulsivity: A review. *Psycholog. Bull.* 1976, 83:1026-1052.

MINDE, K., LEWIN, D., WEISS, G., LAVIGUEUR, H., DOUGLAS, V., and SYKES, E. The hyperactive child in elementary school: A five year, controlled follow-up. *Except. Child.* 1971, 38:214-221.

MORRISON, J. R. and STEWART, M. A. A family study of the hyperactive child syndrome. *Biolog. Psychiat.* 1971, 3:189-195.

NALL, A. Alpha training and the hyperkinetic child—Is it effective? *Acad. Ther.* 1973, 9:5-19.

OFFIR, C. W. A slavish reliance on drugs: Are we pushers for our own children? *Psychol. Today* 1974, 8:49.

PARASKEVOPOULOS, J. and MCCARTHY, J. Behavior patterns of children with special learning disabilities. *Psychol. in the Schools.* 1970, 7:42-46.

POPE, L. Motor activity in brain injured children. *Amer. J. Orthopsychiat.* 1970, 40:783-794.

PUTRE, W., LOFFIO, K., CHOROST, S., and MARX, V. An effectiveness study of a relaxation training tape with hyperactive children. *Behav. Ther.* 8:35-359.

RIE, H., RIE, E., STEWART, S., and AMBUEL, J. Effects of ritalin on underachieving children: A replication. *Amer. J. Orthopsychiat.* 1976, 46:313-322.

RIETH, H. J. A behavioral approach to the management of hyperactive behavior. In M. J. Fine (ed.), *Principles and Techniques of Intervention with Hyperactive Children.* Springfield, Ill.: Charles C Thomas, 1977.

ROGERS, M. E., LILIENFELD, A. M., and PASAMANICK, B. Prenatal and perinatal factors in the development of childhood behavior disorders. *Acta Psychiatrica Scandinavica.* (Suppl. 102) 1955, 1:1-157.

SAFER, D. J. and ALLEN, R. P. *Hyperactive Children: Diagnosis and Management.* Baltimore, Md.: University Park Press, 1975.

SCHMITT, B. D. The hyperactive child. Paper presented at the University of Kansas Medical Center, Kansas City, June, 1974.

SCHMITT, B. D., MARTIN, H. P., NELLHAUS, G., CRAVENS, J., CAMP, B. W., and JORDAN, K. The hyperactive child. *Clin. Pediatrics.* 1973, 12:154-169.

SCHNACKENBERG, B. C. A plea for comprehensive treatment for the hyperkinetic child. *Child Welfare.* 1977, 66:231-237.

SCHRAG, P. and DIVOKY, D. *The Myth of the Hyperactive Child.* New York: Pantheon Books, 1975.

SCHRAGER, J., LINDY, J., HARRISON, S., MCDERMOTT, J., and KILLINS, E. The hyperkinetic child: Some consensually validated behavioral correlates. *Except. Child.* 1966, 32:635-637.

SIMMONS, J. Q. Behavioral management of the hyperactive child. In Cantwell, D. P. (ed.), *The Hyperactive Child: Diagnosis, Management, and Current Research.* New York: Spectrum Publications, 1975.

SOLOMONS, G. Guidelines on the use and medical effects of psychostimulant drugs in therapy. *J. Learning Dis.* 1971, 9:470-475.

SPRAGUE, R. and SLEATOR, E. Methylphenidate in hyperkinetic children: Differences in dose effects on learning and social behavior. *Science.* 1977, 198:1274-1276.

STEWART, M. A. Hyperactive children. *Scientific Amer.* 1970, 222:94-99.

STEWART, M. A. and OLDS, S. W. *Raising a Hyperactive Child.* New York: Harper & Row, 1973.

STRAUSS, A. A. and LEHTINEN, L. E. *Psychopathology and Education of the Brain-Injured Child.* New York: Grune, 1947.

STRAUSS, A. A. and KEPHART, N. C. *Psychopathology and Education of the Brain-Injured Child, II.* New York: Grune, 1947.

SULZBACHER, S. I. Psychotropic medication with children: An evaluation of procedural biases in results of reported studies. *Pediatrics.* 1973, 51:513-517.

THOMAS, A., CHESS, S., and BIRCH, H. G. *Temperament and Behavior Disorders in Children.* New York: New York University Press, 1968.

WALKER, S. Drugging the American child: We're too cavalier about hyperactivity. *Psychol. Today.* 1974, 8:43-48.

WEISS, G., HECHTMAN, L., and PERLMAN, T. Hyperactives as young adults: School, employer, and self-rating scales obtained during ten-year follow-up evaluation. *Amer. J. Orthopsychiat.* 1978, 48:438-445.

WENDER, P. H. *The Hyperactive Child: A Handbook for Parents.* New York: Crown Publishers, 1973.

WERRY, J. S. Developmental hyperactivity. *Pediatrics Clinics of North America.* 1968, 15:581-599.

WILLIAMS, J. I., CRAM, D. M., TAUSING, F. T., and WEBSTER, E. Relative effects of drugs and diet on hyperactive behaviors: An experimental study. *Pediatrics.* 1978, 61:811-817.

WINETT, R. A. and WINKLER, R. C. Current behavior modification in the classroom: Be still, be quiet, be docile. *J. Applied Behav. Analysis.* 1972, 5:499-504.

WUNDERLICH, R. C. Treatment of the hyperactive child. *Acad. Ther.* 1973, 8:375-390.

ZENTALL, S. S. Environmental stimulation model. *Except. Child.* 1977, 43:502-510.

Part II
CASE STUDIES

CHAPTER 2

Behavioral Approaches
To Hyperactivity

While there are conceptual and procedural variations in behavioral approaches, the common denominator is the systematic focus on the behavioral manifestations of the phenomenon being studied. Indeed, for many behaviorists the behavior is the "condition." For other persons, hyperactivity is considered to be an expression of something that is wrong or malfunctioning within the child. Brain damage, maturational lag, or serious psychological disturbance are some of the frequently suspected internal causes of hyperactive behavior. But the behaviorally oriented person is more likely to view the hyperactive behavior as the problem in itself, and to consider the cause and maintenance of the behavior as a function of the reinforcement the behavior is receiving.

Another important element of a behavioral approach is the focus on the present. Key questions posed by behaviorists would include: How is the behavior showing itself now?; Under what conditions does the behavior show itself?; and What can be added or deleted systematically from the contemporary reinforcement picture to potentially affect the behavior? In order to influence the behavior, either events preceding it (stimulus events) or incidents following the behavior (consequent events) will be systematically manipulated and their effects on the behavior studied. Numerous studies have been reported that are supportive of the efficacy of behavioral techniques with hyperactive children (Allen et al., 1967; Allyon et al., 1975; Rieth, 1977; Safer and Allen, 1976; Simmons, 1975).

Behavioral strategies have also been viewed in a broader perspective than just reinforcement of behavior. It has been recognized that a youngster may fail to discriminate between acceptable and unacceptable behavior. Accordingly, some behavioral strategies employed are concerned with helping the child make a more adequate discrimination, and to this end modeling procedures involving live or videotaped models have been used (Nixon, 1969). An additional direction in the application of behavioral principles has been the training of the child to "say things" to himself that can serve as behavioral cues (Meichenbaum, 1977; Kendall, 1977). Research has actually been concerned with the behavioral shaping of cognitive structures as intermediate to the desired behavior change.

One other consideration in the behavior-modification strategies has been the shift from other-controlled to self-controlled procedures. In the early days of developing and implementing behavioral procedures, the focus on exactitude in experimental design, coupled with the emphasis on "the behavior is the thing," removed the client or student from any involvement in his behavior change program. The confluence of several factors, including the concern for rights of children and the recognition that generalization of behavior change often does not occur from one situation to another, has prompted more involvement of children in their own programs. The behavioral area is rich in creativity and variation, and also conveys a basic scientific commitment to operational definition, systematic control, replicability, and verifiability of the treatment.

This brief introduction sets the stage for several detailed case studies. The respective case studies demonstrate the utility of behavioral intervention with children of different ages. Also, the focus of intervention includes both social and academic behaviors. The varied strategies include selective positive reinforcement, contingency contracting, token reinforcement, self-management procedures, and cognitive behavior modification. The settings vary from home to school, and collaborative efforts between parents and professionals are illustrated.

References

ALLEN, K. E., HENKE,, L. B., HARRIS, F. R., BAER, D. M., and REYNOLDS, N. J. Control of hyperactivity by social reinforcement of attending behaviors. *J. Educat. Psychol.* 1967, 56:231-237.

ALLYON, R., LAYMAN, D., and KANDEL, H. J. A behavioral-educational alternative to drug control of hyperactive children. *J. Applied Behav. Analysis.* 1975, 8:137-146.

KENDALL, P. C. On the efficacious use of verbal self-instructional procedures with children. *Cognitive Ther. and Res.* 1977, 1:331-341.

MEICHENBAUM, D. *Cognitive-Behavior Modification: An Integrated Approach.* New York: Plenum, 1977.

NIXON, S. B. Increasing task-oriented behavior. In Krumboltz, J. D. and Thoreson, C. E. (ed.), *Behavioral Counseling.* New York: Holt, Rinehart, & Winston, 1969.

RIETH, H. A behavioral approach to the management of hyperactive behavior. In Fine, M. J. (ed.), *Principles and Techniques of Intervention with Hyperactive Children.* Springfield, Ill.: Charles C Thomas, 1977.

SAFER, D. and ALLEN, R. *Hyperactive Children.* Baltimore, Md.: University Park Press, 1976.

SIMMONS, J. Behavioral management of the hyperactive child. In Cantwell, D. (ed.), *The Hyperactive Child.* New York: Spectrum Publications, 1975.

CASE STUDY #1. THE USE OF SCHOOL AND HOME MANAGEMENT PROGRAMS TO DIMINISH THE INAPPROPRIATE BEHAVIOR EMITTED BY AN EIGHT-YEAR-OLD HYPERACTIVE STUDENT

Herbert J. Rieth

Current Problem

Billy was an eight-year-old, second-grade male student who had a history of being disruptive. He was frequently observed leaving his seat without permission to wander around the classroom in order to visit with friends, and/or to investigate various activities that were being conducted in the classroom. Typically, his movement around the classroom precipitated a commotion, and frequently he became embroiled in altercations with peers. In addition, the teacher reported that Billy would frequently talk out without permission, despite rules and warnings that such behavior was inappropriate. These outbreaks usually disturbed the class and always prompted a reprimand or a consequence from the teacher. Billy's academic work was considered to be average despite his disruptive behavior. The teacher indicated, however, that she thought that his academic performance would improve if he "concentrated" more on paying attention and engaged in less disruptive behavior.

Billy's parents were also concerned about his academic and social behavior. They indicated that he had "always" been a problem because of his refusal to follow requests and directives, altercations with siblings, irritability, and very high activity level. Their current concerns included how to manage his behavior and the inefficacy of medication which had been prescribed for Billy's reported hyperactivity. In addition, his parents were concerned about the appropriateness of their son's school program because of the reported frequency of his inappropriate social behavior, as well as achievement which was not consonant with his "potential."

Background Information

Billy, the first of two children, was born without complications after a full-term pregnancy. His parents indicated that Billy attained all developmental milestones at, or slightly before, the "appropriate" ages. The parents indicated, however, that Billy was always quite active and never required much sleep. Billy's mother recalled that as an infant, he typically slept only a couple of hours at a time and required a considerable amount of holding in order to quell frequent outbursts of crying. As a young child, Billy was always involved in some activity, ranging from dismantling toys to throwing rocks and taunting neighborhood children. He usually moved through these activities in rapid succession. If his parents attempted to entertain him by playing a game with him, Billy typically grew restless after a short period of time. The same behavior characterized his participation while working on home-improvement tasks with his father. His parents reported that his behavior was difficult to manage. They indicated that they set behavioral rules, but Billy was adamant about breaking those regarding throwing items at other children, returning home when called, name-calling, fighting, and destroying property. His parents indicated that they tried "to reason" with Billy. When that failed, they resorted to reprimanding him. In certain cases, he was spanked, sent to his room for an hour, or sent to bed early; with little apparent effect.

As he grew older, Billy's behavior became more resistant to change efforts initiated by his parents. They likened their efforts to trying to contain a tornado. Finally, in exasperation, the parents turned to their pediatrician for assistance. At that time, Billy, who was five years old, was placed on medication to control his "hyperactivity" and to make him more tractable to his parents' management efforts. The parents indicated that they thought the program helped, but they were unable to provide any documenting evidence. They did report, however, that he subsequently reverted to some of his previous behavior patterns.

From his initial enrollment in school until his promotion to second grade, Billy's academic career was characterized as "average" by his teachers, although they unanimously agreed that he appeared to possess "above average" potential. His kindergarten, first-, and second-grade teachers indicated that Billy periodically neglected to submit assignments because they were lost or because they were never completed. In addition, his social behavior required close observation because of his unauthorized movement around the classroom and talking-out without permission. The teachers, however, did not think that there were sufficient grounds to warrant a referral for assessment of Billy's academic and social behavior.

After a parent-teacher conference in November of his second-grade year, Billy's teacher and parents agreed that an evaluation might be beneficial in discovering information that might be used to develop a program to change his behavior. The evaluation was conducted by the school psychologist, and included an *in situ* observation, formal and informal assessment, and analysis of two weeks of assignment papers.

A total of four *in situ* observations were conducted to record the incidence of inappropriate and appropriate behavior, the percentage of time on-task, and teacher-pupil/pupil-pupil interaction patterns. During the initial observations, it was noted that most of Billy's inappropriate social behavior was included in the out-of-seat or talk-out categories. Frequency of these behaviors ranged between three and four per behavior, per 20-minute period. Billy was observed to pay attention an average of 58 percent of the time. It was noted, however, that higher rates of attention occurred in reading than in the other subject areas, and that Billy attended more to independent reading tasks than to written seat-work tasks. Typically, teacher-pupil interactions occurred in conjunction with Billy's emitting inappropriate social behavior. A vast majority of these interactions consisted of reprimands and threats. In a lesser number of cases, Billy was complimented for completing his work or for attending to tasks. Billy's interactions with his peers were minimal, aside from altercations resulting from leaving his desk without permission. Most students tended to avoid him because of his antics.

A series of formal and informal tests were administered. Billy scored in the lower portion of the superior range (IQ > 120) on the Wechsler Intelligence Scale for Children (WISC) and achieved a reading grade-level score of 4.2 and math and spelling grade-level scores of 2.4 on the Wide Range Achievement Test (WRAT). Informal tests in these subject content areas verified these results. Analysis of Billy's papers indicated sloppy work habits, including papers that were never completed or computation problems completed with simple computational errors that could have been corrected had the paper been checked. In other cases, assignments were partially completed, answers were partially crossed out, and holes were erased through pages. The teacher indicated that Billy's "lost" papers were found in his desk, which looked like the wake of a tornado.

Intervention

A twofold intervention was planned, developed, and implemented. One intervention was designed for implementation in school, while the second was designed for implementation in the home. They were not mutually exclusive and were coordinated through the participation of the school psychologist, who was instrumental in designing both interventions.

The classroom intervention focused upon decreasing the number of "talk-outs" and "out-of-seats" emitted by Billy during a 50-minute math period. The class was held from 12:50 to 1:40 every school day. The teacher used event-measurement to record the number of times Billy left his seat without authorization from the teacher and the number of times he talked-out without permission from the teacher. Permission was obtained by raising his hand and requesting permission to leave his seat or talk out. During the five-day baseline, the teacher recorded an average 7.8 talk-outs and 5.2 out-of-seats (see Figure 1). During this condition, the teacher typically scolded Billy for disrupting the class or attempted to ignore him. At the conclusion of the baseline, the teacher had a conference with Billy to talk about his disruptive behavior and attempted to design a reinforcement system to reduce the frequency of disruptive episodes.

The teacher discovered that Billy enjoyed going to the library to pick up and subsequently return audiovisual equipment which was to be used in the classroom on that particular day. Coincidentally, the teacher began scheduling a series of concept-building filmstrips after each math class. In Condition 1, Billy agreed that he would be allowed to pick up and return the filmstrip projector if he did not leave his seat or talk out without permission more than three times during each period. During the five days that this condition was implemented, the mean number of talk-outs was 2.4 and the mean number of out-of-seats was 2.0. The reinforcer was earned on all but one day, when four talk-outs were recorded.

In Condition 3, the criterion for earning the reinforcer was lowered to one talk-out and out-of-seat per period. This condition was in effect for five days, and the mean number of talk-outs was reduced to 1.0 and the mean number of out-of-seats was .20. Billy was able to earn the reinforcer on all but one occasion. Again, after five days, Billy and his teacher conferred regarding his progress and agreed to try a program under which Billy agreed not to talk out or leave his seat without permission during the entire math period in order to earn the opportunity to pick up and return the film-strip projector.

Condition 4 lasted for five days, and during that time Billy averaged .40 talk-outs and .20 out-of-seats per period. He earned the reinforcer on four out of five days.

Upon the completion of this condition, the teacher met with Billy and complimented him again regarding his superlative progress. She asked if he would attempt to maintain this progress without the benefit of the rein-forcement system. He agreed, and the reinforcement contingency was removed. During this three-day condition, the mean number of talk-outs rose to 2.7 and the mean number of out-of-seats increased to 1.7. It is important to note that both behaviors were in accelerating trends when the condition was terminated (see Figure 1).

Immediately after the termination of the reversal condition, the teacher scheduled a conference with Billy to discuss his behavior and the possibility of reinstating Condition 4, where he was required to emit no unauthorized talk-outs or out-of-seats to earn the reinforcer. He readily agreed to par-ticipate in the program. The introduction of the reinforcement program produced immediate reductions in Billy's behavior. The frequency of both behaviors, however, did exceed the frequencies obtained when Condition 4 was in effect previously, but were below the frequencies recorded in the other conditions. Billy earned the reinforcer on two of the four days.

Overall, the teacher was very pleased with the changes in Billy's behav-ior. She indicated that the dimunition of his inappropriate social behavior was accompanied by improvements in his academic performance, partic-ularly in math. Billy was reportedly completing more papers and with greater accuracy. This produced more sources of reinforcement, including his parents. The teacher also indicated that the attitudes of Billy's classmates toward him changed from passivity and avoidance to committed helpfulness. His peers provided reminders regarding classroom rules and praised Billy for behaving appropriately.

The other major facet of the intervention was implemented by Billy's parents. After the assessment was completed, they attended a conference with the psychologist to discuss the results and to plan an intervention. The intervention that was designed included a home-behavior-management

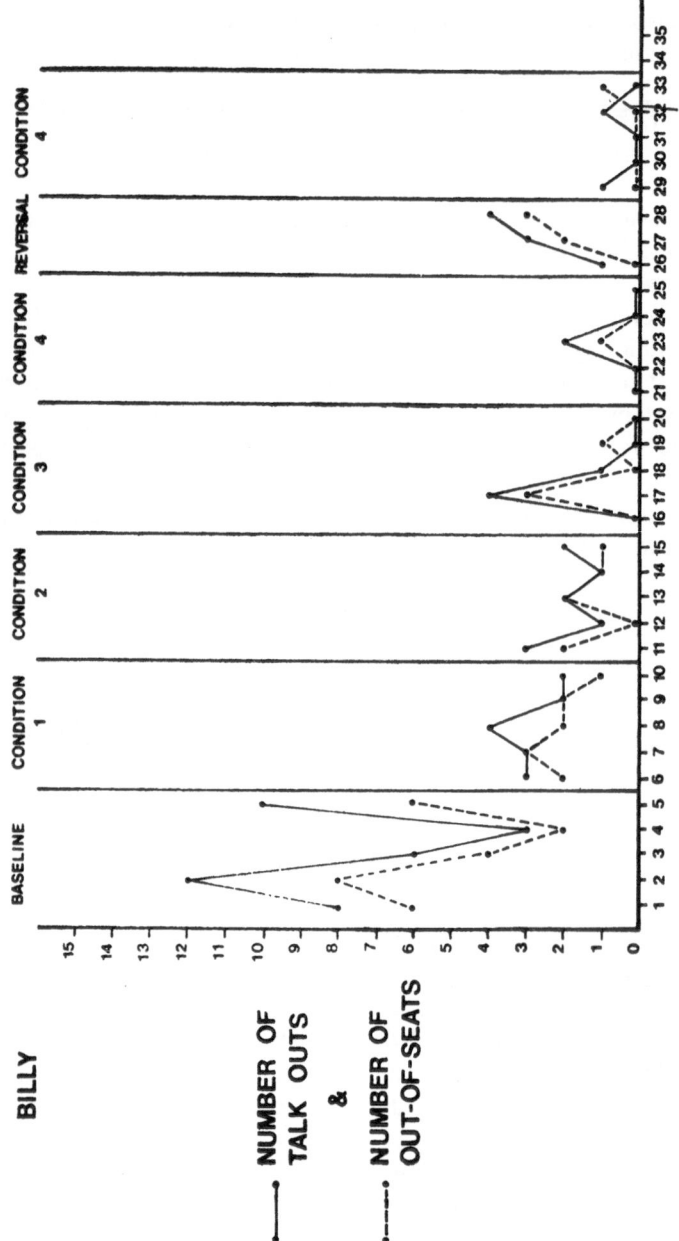

FIGURE 1

program, which included training the parents on how to establish rules; design contingencies; and effectively utilize reinforcement, punishment, and extinction.

Initially, conferences were held to select and define target behaviors for home intervention. The behaviors that the parents selected were adherence to rules (compliance), sibling relations, irritability, and completion of assigned task. The parents first held a conference with their two children to discuss the rules governing behavior in the house, chores assigned, and appropriate interactions. Agreement was reached regarding the definition of appropriate behavior, such as complying with parental requests to return home from playing; arguing with parents, siblings, and peers; care of toys and machinery; and completing assigned chores. The result was an agreed-upon list of appropriate and inappropriate behaviors. The parents used social reinforcement for appropriate behavior and money for the completion of chores, such as cleaning rooms and feeding pets.

Transgressions of the rules were dealt with by using a time-out chair, which was placed in a corner of a low-traffic area of the house. For transgressions, Billy was placed on the chair facing the wall for five minutes. The five minutes commenced when he sat down and became quiet. The parents left the room to minimize the probability of participating in further arguments and checked on him periodically. At the end of the five minutes, a timer buzzer signaled the end of the interval. The parents instructed Billy that once he was placed on the chair, he was not to leave unless they gave him permission; and if he left without permission, he would be given one warning and be spanked for all subsequent episodes. Parental reports indicated marked improvements in behavior due to the use of the reinforcement and punishment system. They also indicated that the allowance system, with public charting for the completion of chores, produced marked improvements in the spontaneous completion of these tasks.

Billy's mother also received instruction on conducting a math tutoring program. Worksheets covering basic addition and subtraction problems were provided. Billy's mother received instructions for using modeling and imitation feedback and reinforcement to conduct intensive, five-minute tutoring sessions daily. In addition, she was encouraged to listen to Billy read periodically in order to reinforce his excellent progress in this area.

The subject of Billy's medication was discussed, and the parents indicated dissatisfaction with its results. They reported that they had discussed this with the physician and he had expressed willingness to terminate the medication. The parents indicated that they refrained from doing this because of their concern regarding their inability to manage Billy's behavior at home and the effects upon his school performance. However, once they began to view the behavioral benefits of the management program, they too indicated a willingness to terminate the medication. Effective day eleven in Figure 1, Billy was removed from medication with his physician's approval. This information was not shared with his teacher initially, in order to ascertain the impact upon his school behavior. The data in Figure 1 indicate that there were apparently no deleterious side effects when the medication was discontinued. Upon termination of the study, the teacher was asked if she had noted any changes in behavior other than those attributable to the system that she had implemented and she answered negatively. She was then apprised that the medication had been discontinued. Parental reports also indicated that there were no deleterious changes in behavior once the medication was terminated.

Conclusion

The case study presented exemplifies the use of coordinated school-home programs that employ behavior-management principles, to reduce the disruptive behavior of an eight-year-old student who was labeled hyperactive. The programs were designed primarily to diminish the incidence of inappropriate behavior in school and in the home. The teacher implemented a management program which afforded Billy the opportunity to pick up and return the audiovisual equipment needed for daily class activities by attaining gradually diminishing criteria of talk-outs and out-of-seat behaviors. The program resulted in greatly diminished frequencies of inappropriate behavior, increased academic productivity, and improved peer relations.

The home program, which was coordinated by a school psychologist, consisted of the provision of behavior-management training for the parents and the cooperative development and implementation of a program designed to reduce inappropriate home behavior and to increase compliance and harmonious interactions. The program employed reinforcement and punishment to successfully reduce the incidence of the noncompliance, arguing, fighting, irritability and activity level, and to increase the frequency of appropriate behavior.

The combination home and school program was found to be sufficiently effective to enable the discontinuance of Billy's medication for hyperactivity without any adverse effects.

CASE STUDY #2. THE USE OF ACTIVITY AND TOKEN REINFORCERS TO INCREASE THE READING ACHIEVEMENT AND APPROPRIATE SOCIAL BEHAVIOR OF A SEVEN-YEAR-OLD HYPERACTIVE STUDENT

Herbert J. Rieth

Jill was a seven-year-old, first-grade pupil who had a history of frequently emitting inappropriate social behavior, a short attention span, and unsatisfactory academic achievement. Despite the teacher directives to desist, Jill frequently talked out without permission, asked irrelevant questions, inquired about other students' activities, and continuously prattled to her teacher and peers about a variety of topics. Another major problem was her unauthorized movement about the classroom: Jill frequently left her seat without permission to wander about the room or to talk with another student. Occasionally, the teacher even observed her crawling about the classroom floor. Jill constantly scanned the room for any sign of activity. Once she observed an event, she would either report on it, ask a question about it, or rush to investigate it.

Jill's academic problems were particularly pronounced in reading. Although she had satisfactory comprehension, the teacher reported that she had difficulty recognizing new words and reading in context. In addition, Jill was easily distracted from her reading and seat-work assignments and the teacher frequently had to redirect her attention to her work, as she often lapsed into talking-out and out-of-seat activities.

The frequency and intensity of Jill's disruptive behavior required the teacher to spend a considerable amount of time attempting to manage her. The teacher employed a variety of management strategies including reprimands, cajolery, praise, and periodic removal to the principal's office. Most of these strategies had transitory effects, however; Jill would attend to assignments or stop misbehaving immediately after being reprimanded, only to soon revert to misbehavior. Consequently, the teacher requested assistance to formulate an intervention for increasing Jill's rate of academic achievement and reducing the frequency of her inappropriate behavior.

Background Information

Jill, the second of three children, was born without complications after a full-term pregnancy. According to reports provided by her parents, all developmental milestones were attained by the appropriate ages. They indicated that Jill was always "very active," "always getting into things," and "quite willful." As a young child, Jill was always busy playing. Confrontations occurred between her and her mother when Jill left the yard without permission; failed to come home when called; or got into altercations with neighbor children and siblings over play activities, possession of toys, and game rules.

Within the home, Jill also frequently argued with her siblings over the selection of TV shows, game rules, dominant roles in play activities, and possession of toys. Jill's mother reprimanded her as the primary mode of managing her inappropriate behavior, although occasional corporal punishment and social isolation were used. The mother reported that Jill always appeared to move rapidly from task to task. The only activity that seemed to maintain her interest for more than 15 minutes was television, which she could watch for a couple of hours at a time. These behavioral patterns persisted until Jill entered school.

In November of her kindergarten year, Jill was referred by her teacher for psychological services. She was concerned about Jill's inability to pay attention and her failure to complete assigned tasks. Because Jill did not listen to directions and because she was always shifting in her seat or moving her seat around her work area, she disturbed other students and failed to complete assignments. These events periodically sparked altercations between Jill and her teacher. The teacher described Jill's work as inappropriate because many assignments were not completed or because they were completed with low accuracy. In many cases, the teacher indicated that Jill began using inappropriate solution strategies and employed those strategies until the assignment was collected.

Group activities, particularly Peabody Language Development activities, also presented problems because Jill did not attend to task and frequently disrupted other members of the group. Although her antics were reprimanded by the teacher, Jill failed to decrease the number of episodes or pay greater attention during those activities. Upon occasion, the teacher would ask Jill to leave the group and return to her seat; but this action was effective until Jill found something else to do. Upon rare occasions, however, Jill would complete an assignment or sit through a lesson and respond appropriately.

The psychologist collected data on the amount on-task talk-outs, and out-of-seat behavior that Jill showed in the classroom and determined IQ and achievement measures. The data indicated that Jill attended to assignments an average of 40 percent of the time. She left her seat an average of five times and talked-out an average of three times per 20-minute observation period. Jill achieved a low average IQ score on the Stanford Binet and scored below grade-level expectations on the Basic Educational

Skills Inventory and the Caldwell Preschool Screening Survey. Jill showed academic weaknesses on items entailing comparison of position (on, off, over, etc.), letter-writing, letter and number identification, and language repertoire.

The psychologist recommended that the teacher increase her social contacts with Jill whenever she caught her paying attention. The teacher was encouraged to visit Jill's work area immediately after assigning work, ask her to repeat the directions, and have her respond to the material while giving her reinforcement and feedback. Other suggestions given the teacher were to make sure that Jill mastered the various academic skills before presenting her with more complex skills, to present only one skill per worksheet, and to provide a weekly review of skills introduced. Wherever possible, the teacher was urged to check Jill's work once during an assignment and again upon completion of an assignment.

The intervention, which the teacher was only partially able to implement, provided reductions in talking-out and out-of-seat behavior and increased attending, academic proficiency, and number of assignments completed. By the end of the year, the teacher reported that although Jill was doing better, her skills hadn't progressed sufficiently to recommend promotion to first grade. Jill's parents agreed with the recommendation; consequently she was retained.

During the next school year, Jill's new teacher expressed concern regarding Jill's academic and social behavior; but conversations with the previous teacher enabled her to successfully implement facets of the previously described program. Overall, the teacher thought that the intervention was effective in managing Jill's social behavior, but she was quite concerned about her student's slow academic progress, her inability to pay attention to academic tasks, and her unwillingness and/or inability to follow directions. Overall, through the use of structure and contingent reinforcement, punishment, and threats, Jill's academic performance was rated below average and her social behavior adequate, and she was passed on to first grade.

Jill's first-grade teacher reported concerns regarding Jill's high-activity level, her short attention span, and her difficulty in learning to read. In the initial months of the school term, the teacher reported that Jill would talk out frequently without permission, often get out of her seat, lie on top of her desk, and crawl around on the floor. Her actions were very disruptive to the entire class, and, because of this nonattending, Jill's academic progress was quite slow. Consequently, the teacher and a consulting psychologist designed a twofold program to reduce or eliminate Jill's inappropriate social behavior and increase her rate of academic achievement.

Intervention

Initially, the academic intervention was implemented during a 15-minute period at the end of the school day when Jill was one of several children who waited approximately 15 minutes for a late school bus. Normally, Jill used this time to get into further trouble. However, one day she approached the teacher and requested help in making sentences from a set of word cards that the teacher had assigned her. Given Jill's overture, the teacher quickly seized the opportunity to work with her.

In order to enable Jill to learn 20 basic vocabulary words selected from her assigned basal text, the teacher presented her with a daily list of 20 words on flashcards. She then recorded the number of words that Jill could correctly identify within three seconds. If Jill could not identify a word, the teacher pronounced it for her, asked her to repeat it. This procedure was repeated during each of the five days of baseline. During this time, Jill correctly identified an average of approximately 13 words per day.

On the sixth day, Jill was told that for each word she correctly identified, she could make a word card which she could take home. The cards were made by writing the target word with a felt-tipped marker on a teacher-supplied blank flashcard. This strategy was implemented for three consecutive days. During this time, Jill correctly identified an average of 18 cards per day.

The teacher instituted a reversal during which she did not allow Jill to use the felt-tipped marker to make word cards to take home. As exemplified by the data in Figure 1, this did not have an impact upon the number of words learned, since Jill continued to learn new words. These data suggested that Jill could continue to acquire new words with periodic teacher praise.

Concurrently, the teacher recorded the percentage of correct responses on daily reading worksheets and reading workbook activities in order to determine if the intervention effects generalized to the student's contextual reading performance. These activities typically involved the student's completing worksheets which entailed using the new vocabulary words in sentences. The data in Figure 2 indicate that when Jill received reinforcement for identifying new words, she typically did better on her daily reading seatwork assignments. Interestingly enough, during the reversal condition, Jill managed to correctly identify all of the vocabulary words correctly but was unable to generalize this knowledge to the worksheets without the benefit of the reinforcer.

Subsequently, Jill was assigned the next reading text in the reading series, while the teacher continued to record the number of new reading vocabulary words correctly identified per day. In addition, the teacher measured the number of talk-outs and out-of-seats that occurred during the two-hour reading period. Talk-outs were defined as speaking out without teacher permission, which was secured by raising the hand. Out-of-seat was defined as being absent from an assigned chair without permission for reasons other than the participation in a reading group, taking completed work papers to the collection basket, or getting a tissue (see Figure 3).

During the four-day baseline period, Jill correctly identified 12 words per day and averaged 3 talk-outs and out-of-seats per class session. When the teacher implemented the reinforcement procedure of allowing Jill to make word cards with a felt-tipped marker for each word correctly identified, the average number of words correctly identified increased to 18 per day and the number of talk-outs and out-of-seats decreased to two per day. When the teacher terminated the reinforcement procedure, the number of words learned per day decreased, but there still was some growth and the number of talk-outs and out-of-seats further declined. As a result of these studies, the teacher reinstated the procedure for reading achievement and reported good success through the remainder of the school year.

Given the success of the previous program, the teacher chose to implement a group-management program during the two-hour reading period. During that time, she recorded the number of talk-outs and out-of-seats occurring in the class during the two-hour observation period. Talk-outs and out-of-seats were defined in the same way as in the previous study, i.e., talk-outs: without teacher permission; and out-of-seats: being absent from an assigned chair for reasons other than participation in a reading group, taking completed work papers to the collection basket, or getting a tissue.

During *Baseline 1,* the teacher recorded an average of 13 talk-outs and out-of-seats during the two-hour period. On day six, each student was given plastic discs to keep on top of his/her desk. During the two-hour reading period, a token was lost for each talk-out or out-of-seat. All students who retained all their tokens during the period earned a Good Worker cover to put on the back of his/her chair and a smiling face stamped opposite the student's name on the Good Worker Chart. The net result, which is depicted in Figure 4, was a reduction in the mean number of talk-outs and out-of-seats to six. Jill averaged only one talk-out or out-of-seat

20 BASIC VOCABULARY IN TIP

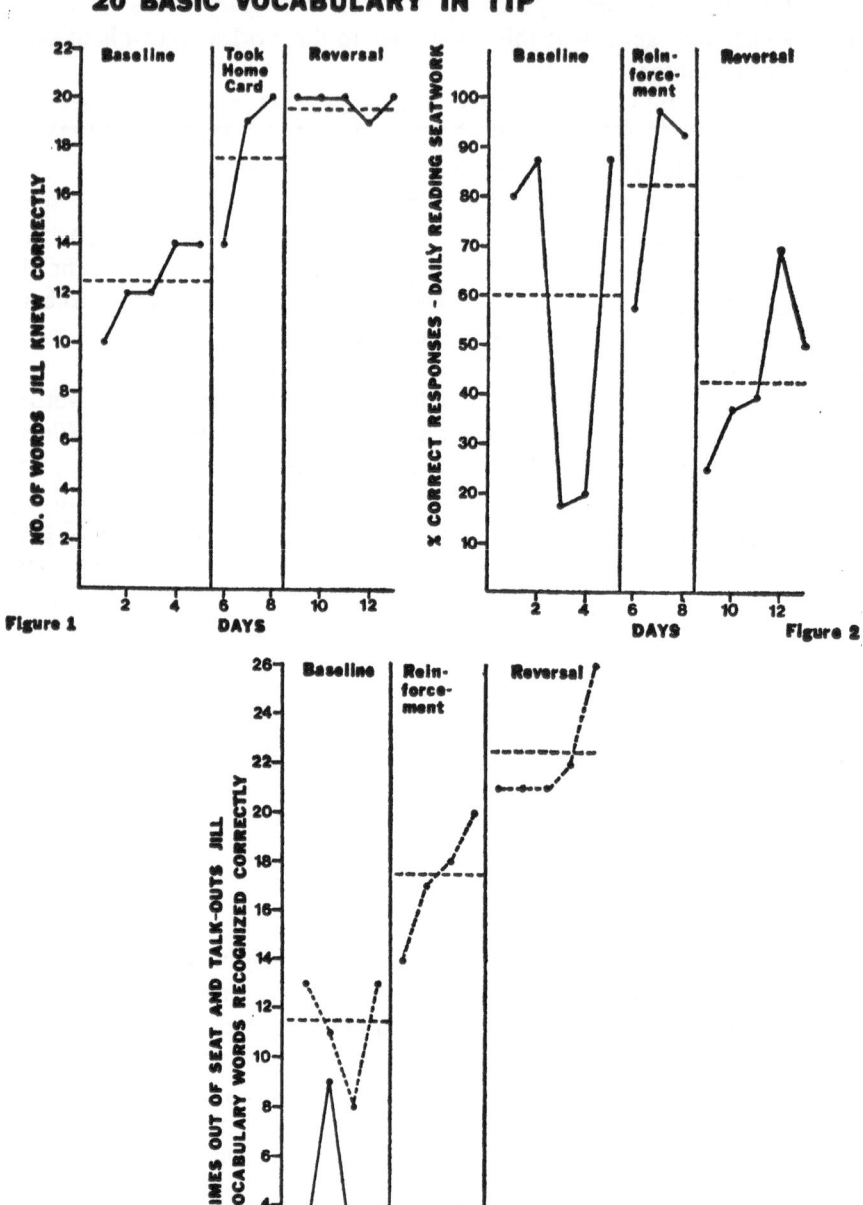

Figure 1

Figure 2

Figure 3

during this condition, as compared with an average of six per day during the baseline condition. When the teacher instituted a reversal and returned to baseline condition, she terminated the Good Worker program and the

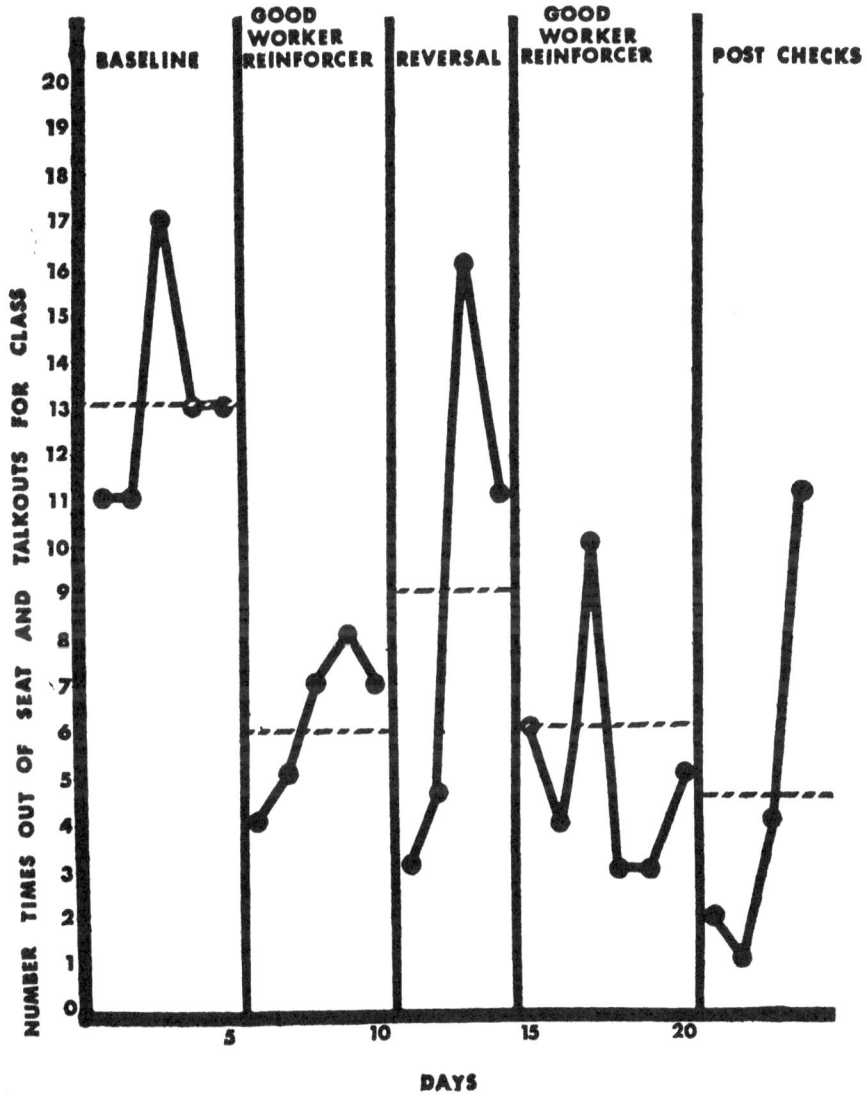

FIGURE 4

class mean number of talk-outs and out-of-seats increased to nine. Jill's total, however, remained stable at one per day.

When the teacher reinstated the Good Worker token program, the mean number of talk-outs or out-of-seats was reduced to six. Jill continued to maintain one talk-out or out-of-seat per period. She maintained this level during the post-check condition, while the class mean decreased further to 4.5 per period.

Overall, this program demonstrated how a practical, low-cost Good Worker token reinforcement program could effectively reduce the number of talk-outs and out-of-seats emitted by a first-grade class and, in particular, by a student who had been labeled hyperactive. The teacher gradually phased out the program and found that Jill's level of appropriate behavior was maintained. The maintenance appeared to be enhanced by the teacher's continuation of the successful academic program which was described previously.

Follow-up information provided by the teacher indicated that the changes were maintained, and Jill attained average grades and was passed to second grade.

In addition to the school program, the parents received assistance from the consulting psychologist in establishing a home-management program. Initially, the program focused upon training the parents, in cooperation with the children, to establish behavioral rules in the home. Once the rules were developed, the parents received assistance in developing lists of consquences for adherence to and noncompliance with the rules. The parents were given specific instruction regarding implementation of the consequences because of their prior reliance on verbal threats, irregular corporal punishments, unsystematic ignoring of inappropriate behavior, and high susceptibility of being manipulated by the children. Instruction focused upon the use of praise and privileges, contingent upon appropriate behavior, and use of time-out from positive reinforcement. The parents were shown how to effectively use a time-out chair, which consisted of placing a chair facing the wall in a low-traffic room or area of a room.

Jill was placed on the chair for predetermined transgressions for five minutes. The time interval was to begin as soon as she sat quietly on the chair. Initially, if she left the chair, she was warned that if she repeated the act, she would be corporally punished and would return to the chair.

After this training, the parents implemented the program. They also received two calls a week from the school psychologist to inquire about the effectiveness of the program, to answer any questions the parents had, and to solve any problems that had arisen.

Once the effectiveness of the program was demonstrated, the number of phone calls was reduced to one per week and ultimately to one every month. Parental reports indicated fewer altercations in the home, greater adherence to rules, and more cooperative play.

It should be noted, however, that this program ran at the same time with both teacher-initiated programs, one of which entailed Jill earning the opportunity to take word cards home. Thus, Jill spent time each evening working on her word cards which somewhat reduced the amount of time she had available to get involved in altercations. Periodically, this set the occasion for appropriate interactions with her parents regarding drill activities over the vocabulary words.

Conclusion

The previous case study described a multifaceted, interrelated program that was developed and implemented for a hyperactive seven-year-old first-grade pupil. The program consisted of multiple interventions implemented by a teacher, in which contingencies were arranged for reading achievement and inappropriate social behavior. The reading program was demonstrated to be effective in increasing Jill's rate of learning new vocabulary and generalized to increased proficiency of reading in context and decreased talk-outs and out-of-seats.

The program was later supplemented by a class-management program which produced further decreased rates of inappropriate behavior and was maintained through the school year.

A home program was developed and implemented concurrently, with comparable success. Jill's parents received assistance in setting up a management program which was successful in reducing levels of inappropriate behavior in the home and increasing levels of appropriate and cooperative behavior.

Thus, the multifaceted, interrelated program was successful in drastically reducing the level of inappropriate behavior of a hyperactive seven-year-old pupil and in increasing the academic performance of the pupil.

CASE STUDY #3. COGNITIVE-BEHAVIOR MODIFICATION IN A CASE OF IMPULSIVITY/OVERACTIVITY*

Philip C. Kendall and A. J. Finch, Jr.

Current Problem

Paul[1] was a nine-year-old white male who was referred to a children's psychiatric facility because of excessive school behavior problems. The teacher had described him as hyperactive, impulsive, and oversensitive to criticism. After having been in the fourth grade for only approximately one month, Paul was demoted back to the third grade because of his inability to function at a fourth grade level. Despite the teacher's efforts, Paul's behavior remained immature and unacceptable. He almost never completed his assignments and was consistently involved in disrupting the class.

Paul was said to not have been liked by his peers who constantly teased him about his size (slight for his age) and his sloppy appearance. He sought attention from anyone who was available, but particularly craved adult attention. Often, he did not play with children of his own age but would instead be found with children who were younger than him. He wandered around frequently seeking attention and was described by his mother as "not respecting authority at all." In summary, Paul's problem was a classroom behavior problem with attention seeking, immaturity, and especially impulsivity/overactivity being the most outstanding characteristics.

Background Information

At the initial intake, a great deal of background information was obtained by a psychiatric social worker during an interview with the mother. Paul was the fourth of five sons born to middle-class parents. Labor was induced at 37 weeks because of erythroblatosis. At birth, Paul weighed 6 lbs., 1 oz. Within several hours following his birth, he became very jaundiced due to Rh factors and his bilirubin level was dangerously high. He received three blood transfusions and apparently made a satisfactory adjustment.

* The preparation of this case-study was supported in part by a University of Minnesota Graduate School Grant (#436 0749 5236 02) awarded to the first author. The material presented in this case study is an expanded and updated version of material formerly published by the present authors in the *Journal of Consulting and Clinical Psychology*. 1976, 44:852-857.

[1] The child's name has been changed to protect his identity.

Paul's mother felt he had always been somewhat developmentally behind her other children, both in size and behavior, and that his manual dexterity was poor. At about one year of age, he was able to stand alone, and he walked at approximately 14 months. By the time he was two-years-old, he was trained for both urine and stool. Paul has been described as not wanting to take time to eat with utensils and apparently considerable conflict has centered around this area. He continued to rush to eat primarily with his hands.

Paul's parents were in marital conflict and, apparently, there had been excessive difficulty for a number of years, with considerable physical fighting between the parents and reported paternal abuse of the children. When Paul was five years of age his parents separated. He remained with his mother and brothers and a number of his mother's "boyfriends," several of whom were live-ins.

When Paul was placed in a day-care center (at the age of four) he was described by his teachers as being very active, immature, and "whiney." At the age of five, he entered kindergarten and, again, his behavior presented extreme problems for him. He was very hyperactive, unable to remain in his seat for extended periods of time, and constantly argued and fought with the other children. Academically, he was relatively slow, with most difficulty being experienced in written work. His school reports were full of comments about his excessive sloppiness and his extremely poor penmanship.

At the end of the third grade, Paul's mother moved to another school system and he entered the fourth grade of a parochial school. Following a few weeks in the fourth grade, the teachers thought that Paul was so far behind academically and emotionally that he was unable to perform at an acceptable level. After a discussion with Paul's mother, it was decided to move him back to the third grade. At this time, his teacher described him as being excessively hyperactive, having his feelings easily hurt, crying excessively, and generally having difficulty getting along with the other children.

Several psychological evaluations had been conducted and indicated that Paul's intellectual functioning was in the low-average to average range. In addition, there had been consistent suggestions of some neurological involvement, and the possibility of a learning disability had been discussed.

Intervention

Prior to the intervention proper, additional assessments were undertaken. These assessments emphasized impulsivity and overactivity—aspects of Paul's behavior that were thought to be central to his current classroom behavior problem. The assessment of cognitive impulsivity used Kagan's (1966) Matching Familiar Figures Test (MFF), whereas the behavioral assessment focused upon recording the number of behavioral "switches." These procedures are described separately below.

Cognitive Evaluation

The MFF is a 12-item match-to-sample task that requires the child to choose the one picture that is identical to a standard from an array of six variants. Average latency to first response and first-response errors were recorded. Based on Paul's MFF means latency (4.59 sec.) and first response errors (nine) he fell into the cognitively impulsive category (i.e. short latencies and high errors in comparison to the MFF performance of other children).

Behavioral Assessment

In an initial meeting, Paul was observed during an interaction with an adult under conditions of no demand. During this assessment session, Paul was moving constantly and rushed from one activity to another. He was frequently out of his chair, talked continuously about multiple topics that made it difficult to follow his conversation, and shifted the direction and apparent purpose of his behavior without observable reason. While playing games, he frequently changed the rules to improve his chances and at times changed the entire game after it had started.

It was decided that the major category of target behaviors to be recorded were the inappropriate and untimely changes or "switches" in Paul's behavior. These switches consisted of Paul's shifting from one behavior to another when the former was not completed. It was decided to record "switches" for three classes of behavior (a) topics of conversation, (b) games played with, and (c) rules of play. For example, a switch in "games played with" was recorded when Paul started to throw darts in the middle of a card game, but not if he started to throw the darts *after* the completion of the card game. Operationally, a switch was recorded when a new or different topic, game, or rule was initiated by the patient when the change did not come at the completion of existing topics, games, or rules.

Baseline observations were obtained in seven ten-minute segments over two sessions, after the initial evaluation session. Paul was not told any specific plans for treatment or what behaviors were going to be worked with. The therapist merely interacted with Paul, following his lead. At the time, the incidences of the target behaviors were recorded (covertly) in such a manner as not to be visible to Paul. Beginning with baseline, a constant array of toys were employed.

Based upon both the MFF data and the observed rate of switching, it was decided that Paul had problems with impulsivity and overactivity and that these should be the central focus of treatment.

Cognitive-Behavioral Procedures

The procedures of the intervention proper employ cognitive and behavioral techniques for treating impulsivity/overactivity. Self-instructional training (Meichenbaum, 1975), modeling (Bandura, 1971), and a response-cost contingency (Kazdin, 1972) are the major components of this cognitive-behavioral treatment (Kendall, 1976, 1977; Kendall and Finch, 1978; in press).

The training in self-instruction began each therapy session. This training was provided along the lines outlined in Table 1.

As can be seen in Table 1, the therapist would first model task performance, instructing himself aloud, having Paul observe. Paul would then perform the task while instructing himself aloud. The therapist and child took turns, with the self instructions fading from overt to covert speech (see sequence of self-instructions in Table 1).

The content of the actual self-instructions were step-by-step verbalizations concerning the problem definition, problem approach, focusing of attention, and coping statements. The coping statements were programed, following a deliberately made mistake by the therapist (e.g., "I should have been more careful and paid closer attention. Well, I can correct it and try again. It's okay."). The coping statements served the purpose of making sure that Paul knew how to deal with a mistake without losing control. It has been observed that many impulsive children become angry or upset after a failure experience and apparently have no means of coping appropriately.

Whenever Paul seemed confused as to his task, he was assisted in employing the verbal self-instructions. Following his familiarization with the general self-instructions, Paul was given practice in the use of individually tailored self-instructions for the specific target behaviors (e.g., switches). For example, with "games" his self-instructions went something like this:

What is it that I'm supposed to remember? I'm to finish playing one game before I begin to play another. I need to keep my mind on what I'm doing and not switch games. When I finish a game I may then play another one.

TABLE 1

Content and Sequence of Self-Instructional Procedures with Impulsive Children. (After Kendall, 1977; Kendall and Finch, 1978, in press; Meichenbaum, 1975, 1977; Meichenbaum and Goodman, 1971)

Content of Self-Instructions		Sequence of Self-Instructions
Problem definition	"Let's see, what am I supposed to do?"	—the therapist models task performance and talks out loud while the child observes;
Problem approach	"Well, I should look this over and try to figure out how to get to the center of the maze."	—the child performs the task, instructing himself out loud; —the therapist models task performance while whispering the self-instructions, followed by
Focusing of attention	"I better look ahead so I don't get trapped."	—the child performing the task, whispering to himself;
Coping statements	"Oh, that path isn't right. If I go that way I'll get stuck. I'll just go back here and try another way."	—the therapist performs the task using covert self-instructions with pauses and behavioral signs of thinking (e.g., stroking beard or chin, raising eyes toward the ceiling);
Self-reinforcement	"Hey, not bad. I really did a good job!"	—the child performs the task using covert self-instructions

During all treatment sessions, Paul was provided with a "training aid"—a card to help him remember to stop and think before responding. This cue card was 5 × 7 inches and was modeled after those employed by Palkes et al. (1968). The instructions to "stop, listen, look and think before I answer" were presented in written and pictorial forms.

The response-cost procedure involved five dimes that Paul was given at the beginning of each session. He was told that these dimes were his to keep, but that he could lose one each time he switched either topic of conversation, games, or rules, depending on the phase of a multiple baseline. Examples were provided until Paul stated that he understood clearly. Whenever an incidence of a switch occurred, a dime was taken and the reason for the loss clearly labeled and explained.

The use of a response-cost contingency is predicated on the fact that impulsive children respond less impulsively under conditions of response-cost than direct reinforcement (see for example Nelson et al., 1975; Errickson et al., 1973). Also, research by Douglas and her colleagues (e.g., Firestone and Douglas, 1975; Parry and Douglas, in press) has unveiled some unique qualities of the hyperactive child's response to reinforcement contingencies. The performance of these children, it appears, is more disrupted by partial and noncontingent reinforcement than that of normals. Also, positive reinforcement attracts the attention of the hyperactive children, distracts them from their task, and orients them toward the rewarding adult. Firestone and Douglas (1975) reported that a reward contingency led to a significant increase in impulsive responding in hyperactive children. These effects suggest that, given the disruptive quality of direct reward, a response-cost procedure may be more desirable.

Consider the following example. A child is given a problem; "What is 6 × 8?" An impulsive child might say "56, uh, 46, no its a 48." Under a contingency where the child receives a reward for the correct answer, the child's fast guessing would have been spuriously rewarded. Response-cost contingencies would prevent fast guessing—when the child said "56" he would lose one chip (reward). The upshot is that impulsive/hyperactive children appear to respond less quickly and more accurately under conditions where they incur a loss for inappropriate responding. Thus, response-cost was utilized in the present case.

The procedure was not, however, response-cost *only*. Rather, the child was given social praise for effort, and was encouraged to self-instruct a reward statement for success. The response-cost contingency was only one part of the treatment and was, in effect, only for errors on the training tasks.

Results

Percentage agreement reliability for the codes observed was determined to be 100 percent. Figure 1 presents the frequency of switchs in topics of conversation, games played with, and rules of play across 10-minute segments of therapy sessions. The baseline number of switches in topics of conversation was relatively high, with the actual frequency ranging from two to six switches per 10-minute segment and a mean of 4.25 switches. Treatment was implemented for switches in topics of conversation in session three, and the incidence of this behavior dropped markedly, while the frequencies of the other behaviors remained relatively constant. For switches in games, the mean during baseline was 4.33 per 10-minute segment and

.12 per segment, following the implementation of treatment for this class of behaviors. Finally, for rules of play, the baseline incidence was 3.31 per segment and, following the implementation of treatment, was reduced greatly.

The use of the multiple baseline design[2] permits an increase in assurance that the obtained results were due to the treatment employed, rather than some source of internal invalidity, since the changes in target behaviors occurred systematically following treatment initiation for that particular behavior. Furthermore, the reliability of the treatment is evidenced by the repeated change that occurred in the rate of target behaviors following treatment. Both the immediacy and the duration of the reduction attest to the strength of the treatmen procedures.

Following treatment, a readministration of the MFF resulted in a mean latency of 18.73 sec. and only five first-response errors. Certainly, these scores suggest a more reflective cognitive style. Furthermore, Paul volunteered his test taking "strategy" following the performance (e.g., "the reason it's this one is cause—see, this one is this way and so is that one") and this strategy was more reflective in nature than his earlier impulsive style.

One of the major concerns was the generalization of the effect of treatment to other settings and other people. Therefore, a test for generalization was built into the design to determine if the appropriate behaviors would generalize. We varied the treatment situation three times. First, we conducted the treatment in a different room. The new room had a different view from the window, various new pieces of furniture, and additional bookshelves. Secondly, we changed the array of toys that had been constant up to this point. Specifically, we introduced several new toys that were desirable to Paul. Finally, we had another therapist administer the program while the original therapist watched and recorded through a one-way mirror.

Support for the generalization of the behavior changes is found in the maintenance of appropriate behavior when the room was changed, the toys varied, and a new therapist was introduced (Figure 1 generalization tests a, b, and c). During these periods Paul was able to control his behavior and maintain the improvement.[3]

In addition to the data gathered during Paul's out-patient visits, we were able to obtain some information from his teachers regarding the nature of

---

[2] See Hersen and Barlow (1976) for a discussion of this and other single-subject designs.

[3] See Kendall (in press) for a discussion of the assessment of generalization in single-subject designs.

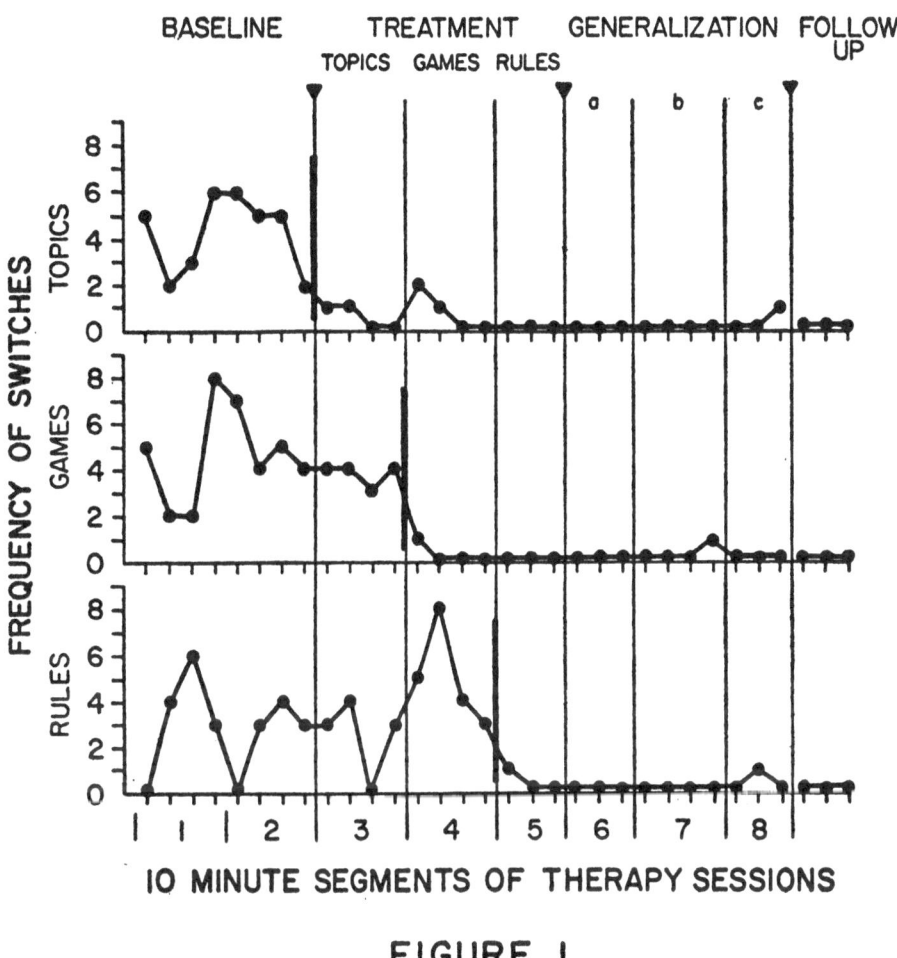

FIGURE I

FIG. 1. Frequency of switches in topics, games, and rules across 10-minute segments of therapy sessions as a function of treatment and generalization tests. Copyright © 1976 by the American Psychological Association. Reprinted by permission.

his behavior in school. This information was unsolicited and recorded on Paul's report card, with the first recording period occurring before Paul came for treatment and the others after treatment began. As can be seen in Table 2, the various categories included the teacher's report of the patient's

TABLE 2

Summary of School Behavior from Report Card*

			Study Skills Category				
Report No.	Listens Attentively	Follows Directions	Completes Work on Time	Works Carefully	Uses Spare Time Well	Begins Promptly	Considerate of Others
1. (pre-treat-ment)	I	S	I	S	I	I	S
2.	S	S	S("better")	S	S("better")	I	S
3.	S	S	S	S	S	S	S
4.	S	S	S	S	S		S

Teachers Overall Comments

1. (pre-treatment)	—not attentive, not participating.
2.	—has been more attentive.
3.	—continues to improve.
4.	—working harder, participates often.

* I and S were the only two grading codes available for use in the reporting of behavior. I = needs improvement; S = satisfactory.

study skills (seven categories) and overall comments for the four report periods. The study-skills categories of "listens attentively," "completes work on time," "uses spare time well," and "begins promptly" all went from I (needs improvement) to S (satisfactory) concomitantly with treatment. Furthermore, the overall teacher comments became more positive, going from "not attentive; not participating" to "has been more attentive" and finally "working harder."

Six months after his formal treatment, Paul was readministered the MFF according to standard instructions. Again, his performance reflects the effectiveness of the treatment program, in that he had a mean latency of 24.7 sec. and only four first-response errors. Likewise, his improvement is reflected in the absence of inappropriate switches during the three ten-minute observation periods (see Figure 1), despite the termination of the specific treatment program six months earlier.

Conclusion

The present case study suggests the potential usefulness of the cognitive-behavioral program in teaching an impulsive, hyperactive youngster to employ verbal self-instructions via modeling, with response-cost for errors as a means of decreasing inappropriate and unacceptable impulsive behaviors. Not only did both latency and error scores on the MFF improve, but there were actual behavioral improvements exhibited during the treatment sessions and behavioral improvements exhibited at school, as reflected by the teacher's comments. Although we acknowledge the important role of the teacher-child relationship in this case, it is felt that the treatment procedures, per se, are essentially responsible for the observed improvements. Nevertheless, additional case studies and group comparison studies are *necessary* to fully understand the most efficacious procedures for the application of the cognitive-behavioral intervention with hyperactive children.

In this regard, several other investigators have reported on both the utility and the potential difficulties of the use of verbal self-instructional procedures, either alone or in combination with other models (e.g. Bornstein and Quevillon, 1976; Bugental et al., 1977; Camp et al., 1977; Douglas et al., 1976; Drummond, 1974; Higa, 1973; Moore and Cole, Note 1; Robertson and Keeley, 1974; Robin et al., 1975; Varni and Henker, in press; Watson and Hall, Note 3). The interested reader is referred to these reports for details.

In a recent review of the evidence for the generalization of the self-instructional procedures (Kendall, Note 4), it was pointed out that, though self-instructional training has been shown to have positive effects on a variety of measures, the results of studies using the combination of cognitive training with behavioral contingency management procedures (e.g. response-cost contingency: see Kendall and Finch, 1978; Kendall and Wilcox, Note 5) have faired somewhat better in the attainment of treatment generalization. Future research efforts should examine the efficacy of the cognitive-plus-behavioral procedures in relation to psychopharmacological treatments. The utility of the cognitive-behavioral approach, as either an adjunct or alternative to medications, merits investigation at this time.

Reference Notes

1. Moore, S. F. and Cole, S. D. *Cognitive Self-Mediation Training with Hyperkinetic Children*. Manuscript submitted for publication, 1977.
2. Robertson, D. and Keeley, S. *Evaluation of Mediational Training Program for Impulsive Children by a Multiple Case Study Design*. Paper presented at the meeting of the American Psychological Association, Montreal, 1974.
3. Watson, D. and Hall, D. *Self-Control of Hyperactivity*. Unpublished manuscript, La Mesa Spring Valley School District, San Diego, California, 1977.
4. Kendall, P. C. *Self-Instructions with Children: An Analysis of the Inconsistent*

Evidence for Treatment Generalization. Manuscript submitted for publication, 1978.

5. KENDALL, P. C. and WILCOX, L. E. *A Cognitive-Behavioral Treatment for Impulsivity: Concrete Versus Conceptual Labeling with Nonself-Controlled Problem Children.* Manuscript submitted for publication, 1978.

References

BANDURA, A. Psychotherapy based upon modeling procedures. In Bergin, A. and Garfield, S. (eds.), *Handbook of Psychotherapy and Behavior Change.* New York: Wiley, 1971.

BORNSTEIN, P. H. and QUEVILLON, R. P. The effects of a self-instructional package on overactive preschool boys. *J. Applied Behav. Analysis.* 1976, 9:179-188.

BUGENTAL, D. B., WHALEN, C. K., and HENKER, B. Causal attributions of hyperactive children and motivational assumptions of two behavioral-change approaches: Evidence for an interactionist position. *Child Dev.* 1977, 48:874-884.

CAMP, B. W., BLOM, G. E., HEBERT, F., and VAN DOORNINCK, W. J. "Think loud": A program for developing self-control in young aggressive boys. *J. Abn. Child Psychol.* 1977, 5:157-169.

DOUGLAS, V. I., PARRY, P., MASTON, P., and GARSON, C. Assessment of a cognitive training program for hyperactive children. *J. Abn. Child Psychol.* 1976, 4:389-410.

DRUMMOND, D. *Self-Instructional Training: An Approach to Disruptive Classroom Behavior.* Unpublished doctoral dissertation, University of Oregon, 1974.

ERRICKSON, E. A., WYNE, M. D., and ROUTH, D. K. A response-cost procedure for reduction of impulsive behavior of academically handicapped children. *J. Abn. Child Psychol.* 1973, 1:350-357.

FIRESTONE, P. and DOUGLAS, V. I. The effects of reward and punishment on reaction times and autonomic activity in hyperactive and normal children. *J. Abn. Child Psychol.* 1975, 3:201-216.

HERSEN, M. and BARLOW, D. H. *Single Case Experimental Designs.* New York: Pergamon, 1976.

HIGA, W. R. *Self-Instructional Versus Direct Training in Modifying Children's Impulsive Behavior.* Unpublished doctoral dissertation, University of Hawaii, 1973.

KAGAN, J. Reflection-impulsivity: The generality and dynamics of conceptual tempo. *J. Abn. Psychol.* 1966, 71:17-24.

KAZDIN, A. E. Response cost: The removal of conditioned reinforcers for therapeutic change. *Behav. Ther.* 1972, 3:533-546.

KENDALL, P. C. (Producer). A cognitive-behavioral treatment for impulsivity. Minneapolis: University of Minnesota, 1976. (Film)

KENDALL, P. C. On the efficacious use of verbal self-instructional procedures with children. *Cognitive Ther. and Res.* 1977, 1:331-341.

KENDALL, P. C. Assessing generalization (transfer) and the single-subject strategies. *Behav. Ther.* in press.

KENDALL, P. C. and FINCH, A. J. A cognitive-behavioral treatment for impulse control: A case study. *J. Consulting and Clin. Psychol.* 1976, 44:852-857.

KENDALL, P. C. and FINCH, A. J. A cognitive-behavioral treatment for impulsivity:

A group comparison study. *J. Consulting and Clin. Psychol.* 1978, 46:110-118.

KENDALL, P. C. and FINCH, A. J. Developing nonimpulsive behavior in children's cognitive-behavioral strategies for self-control. In Kendall, P. and Hollon, S. (eds.), *Cognitive-Behavioral Interventions: Theory, Research, and Procedures.* New York: Academic Press, in press.

MEICHENBAUM, D. Self-instructional methods. In Kanfer, F. and Goldstein, A. (eds), *Helping People Change.* New York: Pergamon Press, 1975.

MEICHENBAUM, D. *Cognitive-Behavior Modification: An Integrative Approach.* New York: Plenum, 1977.

MEICHENBAUM, D. and GOODMAN, J. Training impulsive children to talk to themselves: A means of developing slef-control. *J. Abn. Psychol.* 1971, 77:115-126.

NELSON, W. M., FINCH, A. J., JR., and HOOKE, J. F. Effects of reinforcement and response-cost on cognitive style in emotionally disturbed boys. *J. Abn. Psychol.* 1975, 84:426-428.

PALKES, H., STEWART, W., and KAHANA, B. Porteus maze performance of hyperactive boys after training in self-directed verbal commands. *Child Dev.* 1968, 39:817-826.

PARRY, P. and DOUGLAS, V. I. The effect of reward on the performance of hyperactive children. *J. Abn. Child Psychol.* In press.

ROBIN, A. L., ARNEL, S., and O'LEARY, K. D. The effects of self-instruction on writing deficiencies. *Behav. Ther.* 1975, 6:178-187.

VARNI, J. and HENKER, B. A self-regulation approach to the treatment of the hypertive child. *Behav. Ther.* In press.

CASE STUDY #4. THE USE OF SELF-MANAGEMENT TO IMPROVE READING SKILLS IN A HYPERACTIVE CHILD

A. Lee Parks and R. L. Sherbenou

Current Problem

Charles was an eight-year, three-month-old second-grade boy who had a history of hyperactivity. He was very active both in class and on the playground, and he occasionally fought with his peers. Prior to the study, he had received Ritalin for about two years. Throughout the study, he received no medication. His listening skills were excellent, but his reading was very poor. His reading level was judged to be on kindergarten level, since he knew only one word (dog) on a pre-test on the Dolche Word List. Both fine and gross motor skills were considered to be normal or better.

Background Information

Charles' early developmental history is not known. He had no sibling for about six years. His parents were divorced when he was about four to six years old. After about two years, his mother remarried. At the time of the study, Charles had a two-year old sister. He seemed to have an active role with his stepfather.

Charles had been retained in the first grade; his present teacher received him at the beginning of the second grade. His school history was marked by fidgeting, inattention to lessons, and moving around the room.

Intervention

The program was developed by a consulting psychologist and the classroom teacher. Word recognition was selected as the target behavior. It was felt that Charles had the potential capability for learning to read, if his over-activity could be constructively channeled. Thus, activity itself was not seen as a problem, but rather what was done with that activity. This study reports the results of a self-managed motivational system for learning sight-words.

Each day, Charles received ten words which were handwritten and auditorally recorded on Language Master cards. These words were those that Charles was unable to sight read within 20 seconds on the pre-test. No word was used on more than one day.

The design of the study had three basic phases: (1) no reinforcement; (2) self-reinforcement; and (3) teacher-management of reinforcement.

The following procedures were used in all phases. Seated before a Language Master, Charles picked up his stack of ten Language Master cards containing the day's new words. He would (1) run each card through the machine to hear the word, (2) write the word on a piece of paper, and (3) repeat the process for each card two times. Fifteen minutes were allowed for this process and were referred to as the "teaching time." Charles tested himself on the list of words immediately after the teaching time, because it was found that he had almost no ability to retain the words for any length of time.

The test was self-administered in the following way: (1) Charles looked at the word to determine if he knew it, (2) he then auditorially recorded his response on the Language Master card and moved to the next word, and (3) after he had responded to all of the words, he checked his answers against the correct ones by listening to them on the Language Master cards. Ten minutes were allowed for testing time each day. Cheating was prevented by taping the correct feedback lever down, which prevented Charles from hearing the correct word spoken by the teacher. When Charles was ready to check his responses, the teacher untaped the auditory feedback lever.

Baseline 1

During Baseline 1, Charles worked through his list of words, reporting to the teacher the number he got correct. No special consequences were provided. In a matter-of-fact manner, the teacher reported the number of new words learned and asked Charles to return to his other work. That is, she purposely tried to be neutral, minimizing the possibility of social reinforcement. She always double-checked the reported number correct with Charles' recorded response on the Language Master cards.

Self-reinforcement. During the self-reinforcement phase, Charles was provided with the materials needed in order to reinforce himself. He was given two metal rings; one ring had ten plastic tabs hooked to it and the other ring was empty. Charles was given the following instructions when introduced to the self-reinforcement procedure: "Here are some tokens. Each time you get a word correct on your test, I want you to take a token off this ring and put it on yours. With the tokens you earn you will be able to buy things. You may use them to buy art supplies, getting to be first in line, getting to be a P.E. leader, and other things. Remember, each time you get a word correct, you should take a token and put it on your ring." During each day of this phase Charles was able to give himself tokens for words correctly recalled at testing time.

Baseline 2

During this phase, conditions were changed from self-reinforcement to no reinforcement. Charles was told that he had been doing so well, that it was felt that he did not need the tokens anymore. He followed all the usual procedures, except that he received no tokens for words correctly recalled.

Teacher-managed reinforcement. Following Baseline 2, a teacher-managed reinforcement phase was initiated. Charles was given the following instructions: "Here are some tokens. Each time you get a word correct on your test, I will give you a token from this ring and put it on yours. With the tokens you earn you will be able to buy things like you did before." During the testing period, the teacher stood beside Charles and dispensed a token saying "Very good" each time he correctly responded to the word printed on the card.

Reliability of measurement. Reliability for word-recognition performance was assured by having the teacher listen to Charles' recorded responses. Thus, the teacher always compared his recorded responses with the number of words correctly recorded on the Language Master cards. The teacher's count was the number of correct responses plotted, not the child's count.

Inter-observer reliability on cheating behavior was obtained by having the experimenter and the teacher independently observe Charles as he worked during the testing time. They watched for any instances in which he gave himself a token when he had not verbally recorded the correct response.

There were no instances found in which Charles reported that he had learned more words than he actually had. Inter-observer reliability on noncontingent self-reinforcement, "cheating," was always 100 percent since neither observer ever noted such behavior.

Results

Figure 1 is a graph of Charles' word recognition. His median word-recognition rate during the Baseline 1 was 30 percent. Two weeks of data not presented in Figure 3 show that the baseline is stable, not ascending. Instituting self-reinforcement produced as immediate increase in percent of words recognized. The median rate during this phase was 60 percent.

As the rates continued to decrease during the self-reinforcement phase, it was decided that no tokens were to be kept unless Charles earned a minimum numbr for that particular session. This requirement remained in effect throughout this phase and the teacher-managed reinforcement phase also. He was required to earn five per session before being allowed to keep any. This was done because it seemed as though Charles would quit trying after he had earned a small amount of tokens. Inspection of the graph shows

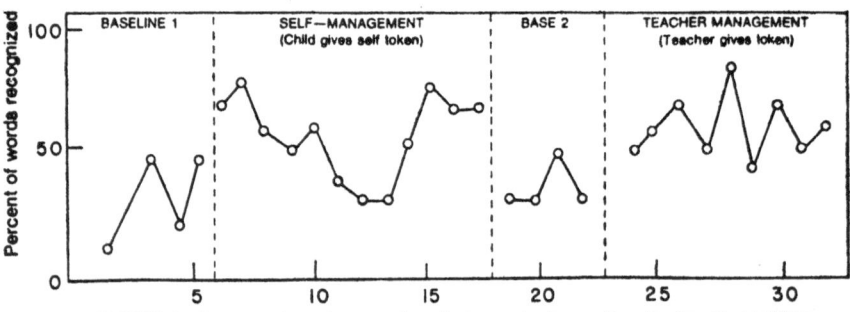

FIGURE 1: Percent of words correct each day under the various treatment conditions.

the point at which this was done. It may be seen that his performance dramatically increased.

Return to Baseline 2 produced a noticeable drop in word recognition to a median rate of 30 percent.

When conditions were changed from Baseline 2 to Teacher-managed Reinforcement, the percent of words correctly recalled increased to a median rate of 60 percent.

Conclusion

The results of this study show that this particular hyperactive child was able to contingently administer tokens to himself for words correctly recalled. Self-administration of tokens resulted in an increase in performance over the previous baseline rate. When the token system was eliminated, the child's performance decreased to a level very much like the original baseline rate. Upon reinstating the token system, teacher-administered, performance increased to a level similar to that obtained during the previous self-management condition.

Although no direct measures were taken of Charles' hyperactivity, the teacher reported that his behavior during the self- and teacher-management conditions was dramatically different from the usual. Reading period had been a particularly difficult time for Charles. He was inattentive to his lessons, tipping backward on his chair, talking to others, moving about the room, and generally fidgeting. During the reinforcement phases of this study, there were almost no such instances of this behavior. This observation was confirmed by the experimenter.

These results suggest that there is reason to expect that some hyperactive children may be able to manage their own academic performance. If a young hyperactive child can effectively assist in the management of his own academic performance, it may be more likely that older children will also be able to do so. Subjective reports by the teacher indicated that hyperactivity ceased to be a problem during reinforcement phases. From these results, it is expected that self-management of reinforcement could be a useful technique for other young hyperactive children.

CASE #5. EFFECTS OF PARENT TRAINING ON BEHAVIORAL TEMPO IN A PRESCHOOL-AGED BOY

Mary Mira and Chris Milar

Elevated behavioral tempo, particularly of behavior that is annoying to adults, brings many parents to treatment facilities for help for their children. Many of these children display clusters of behaviors of similar topography, leading to descriptions of "hyperactive" (Patterson, 1974) or "deviant" (Lobitz and Johnson, 1975). These behaviors share the characteristic of being highly aversive to adults, and include demanding or commanding statements to adults, frequent activity changes, high rates of motor behavior, "smart talk," interrupting, violations of rules, and noncompliance.

Recently there have been several studies concerning how parents interact with these children, whose higher-than-tolerable rates of deviant behavior bring them to treatment. A consistent finding is that the parents themselves display higher-than-normal rates of certain behaviors, such as commands, questions, criticisms, and other directive comments; and respond to a greater proportion of their children's total behavior, than do parents of normals. Lobitz and Johnson (1975) found that parents of children referred for treatment for deviant behavior were more controlling, used more negative comments and consequences, and issued more commands than parents of nonreferred children. These parents were also more negative to nondeviant as well as deviant behavior than were parents of normals.

Johnson et al. (1973) looked at parental responses to deviant and nondeviant behaviors in normal children. They found that the more deviant of these children received more attention from parents for deviant acts than did low-deviant children for similar behaviors. These more deviant, normal children also received more attention for positive behaviors. Forehand and Scarboro (1975) also found that in a structured play situation, between normal children and their mothers, an increase in number of commands from the mother accelerated the children's oppositional behavior. Similarly, Johnson and Lobitz (1974) found that parents could manipulate the level of deviancy in their normal children when instructed to make their children "look bad," and that they did so by increasing the frequency of commands and negative responses to them. The effect of accelerated parental commands was an increase in the frequency of deviant behavior.

It is possible, that the high rate of directive behavior of parents is reactive; that parents respond to their perceived lack of control over the form and tempo of the child's behavior by accelerating their commands and questions. This hypothesis is supported by findings such as those of

Terdal et al. (1976), who studied interactive behaviors of mothers and their developmentally delayed children. They found that when children's feedback to parents was inadequate, inadequacy being defined as no response or inadequate responding, the result was an increase in directiveness on the part of mothers. However, the outcome of increased parental directiveness among children with deviant behavior is generally not increased control over the interaction or over their children's behavior, and it is at this point that parents seek help for the problem. Fortunately, deviant behavioral tempo can be altered by intervening in the way in which parents respond to it (Daniels, 1973; Frazier and Schneider, 1975). The same success has been reported in the classroom (Patterson et al., 1965; Rieth, 1977).

In the case study which follows, the deviant behavioral tempo of a child is modified by systematically altering the differential frequency of two classes of maternal comments: (a) attending and praising statements, (b) commands and questions; plus the introduction of a simple punishment procedure. Althuogh this procedure has been successful for the treatment of deviant child behavior (Forehand and King, 1977; Peed et al., 1977), its impact on behavioral tempo is not elsewhere reported.

Current Problem

Kevin is a three-year-old boy referred to an interdisciplinary developmental disabilities clinic by his mother, who was an acquaintance of a staff member. The mother described Kevin as having discipline and emotional problems, with hyperactivity and temper tantrums being the prominent features. She described herself as being at "wit's end," due to his behavior; she felt that he was not developing normally in his ability to understand what she wanted him to do.

Upon initial screening, it was apparent that Kevin had no developmental problems; that he was a bright, highly active child with good verbal and coordination skills.

The assessment of the problem behavior was carried out in the clinic setting in two play situations, in which the interaction between Kevin and his mother was observed through a one-way mirror. In the first condition, which was a free-play arrangement, the mother was instructed to play with Kevin for ten minutes, allowing him to select any of the toys in the room he chose to play with. She was not to direct the play, but merely to follow his lead in the activities. This was followed by a 10-minute structured-play condition, in which the mother directed the play, determining which toys they would use and in which sequence.

During the free-play situation, in spite of instructions to the contrary, his mother's primary way of interacting with Kevin was by asking him many questions. She did this more than four times per minute. She also gave him commands more than once per minute. Her comments about his play, or feedback to him that he was doing well, occurred only about twice per minute. Kevin moved from one activity to another, responding to only one fourth of his mother's instructions.

In the structured-play situation, when asked to assume control of the play, the mother accelerated the frequency of her commands to more than seven per minute, and asked questions 2½ times per minute. She met Kevin's obvious lack of compliance (he responded appropriately to only five percent of her instructions) by repeating her commands many times. Kevin responded to his mother's repeated commands with verbal bargaining, ignoring her, tantrums, and destruction of the toys. It was clear that Kevin's mother needed to improve her control over both the form and the tempo of his behavior. The starting point for this needed to be improvement of her ability to attend to and follow along with his appropriate behavior. She would then need to improve the clarity and directness of her instructions, while reducing their over-all rate; learn a more effective way of dealing with his deviant responses; and then apply all of these skills to the task of altering the tempo of Kevin's behavior.

Background Information

Kevin was the product of a normal pregnancy and delivery. His early history and development were unremarkable. He achieved developmental landmarks, including speech, at the expected times. Regarding the onset of the behavior problems, his mother reported only that he had always been hard for her to manage.

Kevin was the only child in the home. His parents were divorced a year before the referral. His father alternated his residence between the local community and overseas, so Kevin spent time with him on an irregular basis. Kevin did not attend a preschool, but was cared for by a baby-sitter while his mother worked part-time. She had not previously sought help for Kevin, except to discuss his difficulties with his pediatrician, who concurred with her decision to seek help.

Intervention

The strategy of treatment was to bring Kevin's behavioral tempo more under the control of his mother and those events that she could identify and manipulate, and less under the whimsical control of setting events. Once this was accomplished, his mother would then be in a better position to work directly on those behaviors which were occurring at unacceptably high rates. The training program for the mother was designed to teach her alternate ways of interacting with Kevin. The specific treatment goals for her included: (a) reducing the frequency of her questions and repeated commands, particularly in those situations when it was not necessary for her to direct his activities; (b) increasing her use of descriptive attending statements, praise, and nonverbal cues of approval when his behavior was appropriate; and (c) teaching her a simple warning and time-out method to insure compliance with her instructions.

The first three weekly sessions were spent training the mother to improve her skills of attending to Kevin and praising him for appropriate behavior, using only the unstructured-play situations. For the first five minutes of each session, the mother played with Kevin while the therapist observed and recorded remotely. The remainder of the session was devoted to giving the mother feedback about her behavior, modeling by the therapist, role playing by the mother, and practice by the mother with Kevin. She was taught specifically to restrict herself to praising his behavior, describing what he was doing or describing the objects he was using. She was to avoid all questions and commands in this situation, except for those initial statements necessary to structure the situation for Kevin. She also practiced these skills in a daily home-play session of 15 minutes. This phase of treatment continued until Kevin's mother was able to follow his play with praise and attending statements at a combined rate of ten per minute, with an absence of questions or commands.

The reason for the initial emphasis on teaching attending and praising skills was to give the mother a set of responses for appropriate behavior that would differ markedly from responses to behavior that was unacceptable in either rate or form. Increased differentiation in parental responding would help Kevin differentiate between acceptable and unacceptable behavior.

At the fourth session, the mother was introduced to the control procedures through a structured-play situation which was to direct. She was taught to use commands which were simple, imperative sentences that communicated precisely what was to be done. If Kevin did not begin to comply within five seconds, he was given a warning that he would be placed in the corner if he did not do what he was told. If he still did not comply within five seconds, he was matter-of-factly taken to a chair in the corner and required to remain there until he was quiet for two minutes. If he left the chair, he was given a warning and failure to heed the warning resulted in two firm swats on the seat administered by the mother. Again, these skills were taught by verbal description, modeling by the therapist, role playing, and practice.

The mother was instructed that following this session she was to begin using direct commands, warnings, and time-out for noncompliance in the home. The mother kept records of the frequency of warnings, time-outs, and the circumstances in the home. The home applications was closely supervised by visits by the therapist. In addition, the mother was given directions for generalization of the procedures to settings outside the home. This phase of the training program lasted for three weekly sessions, by which time the mother was using the procedures correctly; she demonstrated good control and pacing of Kevin's activities and his compliance was virtually 100 percent.

Changes in Kevin's Behavior Over the Treatment Sessions

Compliance. The most powerful impact of the program on Kevin's behavior was its effect on his compliance to his mother's instructions. During the baseline session, he complied with 25 percent of her commands in a free-play situation and only five percent in the structured format. By the sixth session, Kevin's compliance was 100 percent in the strucutred-play setting and nearly 100 percent to naturaly occurring instructions in the home. Kevin's mother used his increased willingness to obey to modify the tempo of his behavior. During the structured-play practice sessions in the clinic and in the daily activities in the home, she could alter his tempo by carefully pacing her instructions and by using specific cues which were now functional to reduce activity level; such as "wait," "sit down," and "keep your hands in your lap." An indication of the impact of her control on his activity level is the fact that during the structured-play segment of the fifth treatment session, Kevin did not once cross into a new quadrant of the room; whereas his frequency had been as high as three times a minute in the first session.

Behavioral tempo. Since the parent-training sessions were video recorded, it was possible to review the tapes and record a number of the child's behaviors. Those which were selected as components of his overactivity included shifts from one activity to another, changes in body position, movement around the room, and interrupting adult conversation. Each of the treatment sessions included three types of situations: (a) free play between mother and Kevin, (b) structured play, and (c) conversation between parent and therapist while the child played independently. His activity in this last type of situation was used as the measure, since it more closely approximated out-of-clinic settings and in essence represented a generalization to a condition in which the mother was not exercising direct control.

An activity shift was recorded each time Kevin abandoned one class of objects that he was relating in play, or one activity for another. During the initial parent-training session, the rate with which he changed from one activity to another during those minutes when the mother was not interacting directly with him was 1.9 per minute. The rate declined to .4 per minute by the last session.

A position shift was recorded each time Kevin changed from sitting to standing or kneeling. This behavior also declined over the sessions from 1.9 per minute to .7 per minute.

To measure movement around the room, the treatment space was considered to be blocked off into four quadrants. At the start of the program, Kevin crossed a quadrant boundary 2.97 times per minute and declined systematically to .26 per minute by the end of treatment.

Interruptions were recorded each time that Kevin directed a question to one of the adults or made statements requesting their attention while mother and therapist were talking. Initially, his occurred 1.3 times a minute; declining to .4 per minute during the last session.

If only these five behaviors are considered together, at the start of the program Kevin either moved his body, talked out, or changed activity eight times a minute. Such a rate over a sustained period would undoubtedly result in any child's activity level being noted and perhaps labeled as deviant by adults. This total activity rate declined to 1.69 per minute at the end of the program.

Conclusion

Kevin's mother was able to influence his behavioral tempo and reduce the frequency of his undesirable behavior by modifying the frequency of some of her interactional responses. In a free-play situation, she was able to use selective attention, in the form of descriptions of his activity and praise, to pace his behavior at an acceptable tempo. In a structured situation, as well as in daily home activities, she could control the form and pace of his behavior by using the attending and praising skills and instructions which were direct, simple, nonrepetitive, and backed up by a simple warning and time-out procedure.

References

DANIELS, L. K. Parental treatment of hyperactivity in a child with ulcerative colitis. *J. Behav. Ther. and Exp. Psychiat.* 1973, 4:1-2.

FOREHAND, R. and KING, H. E. Noncompliant children: Effects of parent training on behavior and attitude change. *Behav. Modif.* 1977, 1:93-108.

FOREHAND, R. and SCARBORO, M. E. An analysis of children's oppositional behavior. *J. Abnorm. Child Psychol.* 1975, 3:27-31.

FRAZIER, J. R. and SCHNEIDER, H. Parental management of inappropriate hyperactivity in a young retarded child. *J. Behav. Ther. and Exp. Psychiat.* 1975, 6: 246-247.

JOHNSON, S. M. and LOBITZ, G. K. Parental manipulation of child behavior in home observations. *J. Applied Behav. Anal.* 1974, 7:23-31.

JOHNSON, S. M., WAHL, G., MARTIN, S., and JOHANSSON, S. How deviant is the normal child? A behavioral analysis of the preschool child and his family. In Rubin, R. D., Brady, J. P., and Henderson, J. D. (eds.), *Advances in Behavior Therapy.* Vol. 4. New York: Academic Press, 1973.

LOBITZ, G. K. and JOHNSON, S. M. Normal vs. deviant children: A multi-method comparison. *J. Abnorm. Child Psychol.* 1975, 3:353-374.

PATTERSON, G. R. An empirical approach to the classification of disturbed children. *J. Clin. Psychol.* 1964, 20:326-337.

PATTERSON, G. R., JONES, R., WHITTIER, J., and WRIGHT, M. A. A behavior modification technique for the hyperactive child. *Behav. Res. Ther.* 1965, 2:217-226.

PEED, S., ROBERTS, M., and FOREHAND, R. Evaluation of the effectiveness of a standardized parent training program in altering the interaction of mothers and their noncompliant children. *Behav. Modif.* 1977, 1:323-350.

RIETH, H. J. A behavioral approach to the management of hyperactive behavior. In Fine, M. J. (ed.), *Principles and Techniques of Intervention with Hyperactive Children.* Springfield, Ill.: Charles C Thomas, 1977.

TERDAL, L., JACKSON, R. H., and GARNER, A. M. Mother-child interactions: A comparison between normal and developmentally delayed groups. In Mash, E. J., Hamerlynck, L. A., and Handy, L. C. (eds.), *Behavior Modification and Families.* New York: Brunner/Mazel, 1976.

CASE STUDY #6. CONTINGENCY CONTRACTING WITH A HYPERACTIVE BOY AND HIS PARENTS*

Joan E. Backman, H. Bruce Ferguson, and Ronald L. Trites

Current Problem

Chris B. was an eight-year-old boy referred to the Neuropsychology Laboratory of the Royal Ottawa Hospital because of his disruptive and hyperactive behavior at home and at school. The most troublesome behavior problem at home was Chris' temper tantrums, which occurred several times each day. In addition, his parents expressed concern that Chris was not fulfilling any responsibilities around the house and failed to comply with their requests to do so. During an interview with his grade-three teacher, it was reported that Chris was extremely restless and inattentive. However, his teacher felt that despite these difficulties he had made considerable academic and social progress during the school year.

Background Information

Chris B. lived at home with both parents and his three-year-old brother. He had been a full-term baby, and the pregnancy and delivery were reported to have been uneventful. All developmental milestones occurred within normal limits. Chris' medical history showed two instances of high fever associated with respiratory infections, but he had no current medical problems. He had never been administered stimulant medication.

His parents reported that he had always been a "difficult" child, tending to over-react to change and to be very active. His younger brother, on the other hand, was perceived by them to be a quiet and happy child. His father felt that Chris' behavior problems were of "biological" origin, and was skeptical about Chris' ability to control his actions and emotions, particularly his temper tantrums. He reported that he had been "hyperactive" as a child.

A neuropsychological examination at age seven years, six months consisted of language, perceptual, IQ, and academic achievement tests, along with a standardized motor and sensory examination. Chris obtained a Verbal IQ of 104, a Performance IQ of 85, and a Full Scale IQ of 94 on the Revised Wechsler Intelligence Scale for Children. Academic achieve-

* This project was supported by a grant (#6606-1237-44) from the Health Programs Branch, Health and Welfare Canada to R. L. Trites and H. B. Ferguson.

ment testing indicated that reading and arithmetic functions were at the early grade-two level. Performance levels on motor and sensory tasks were within normal limits. Personality testing and Conners' parent and teacher rating scales indicated that Chris was impulsive, inattentive, and very active, particularly in school. Thus, Chris was physically well-developed, well coordinated and possessed average learning capability. There was no evidence of cerebral dysfunction and he was seen to be a moderately hyperactive youngster whose school progress was lagging slightly as a result of his inattentive and disruptive behavior.

Intervention

Contingency contracting was selected as an appropriate intervention strategy with this family. This technique involves the negotiation and writing of a contract between the child and his parents, explicitly detailing what behaviors are expected of the child, and what rewards or sanctions will be delivered from his parents contingent upon his behavior. Typically, the parents and/or child record points earned and taken away on a tally sheet, and reinforcement is delayed until sufficient points have been accumulated. This technique was pioneered by Homme et al. (1969) for use in the classroom. Stuart (1971) and Stuart et al. (1976) subsequently used contingency contracting to modify the home behaviors of delinquent adolescents. Sixty youths were randomly assigned to either a contracting group or a placebo treatment group consisting of periodic therapist contact without active intervention. Dependent measures included ratings by both parents and a recording of juvenile court contacts. Results indicated that the contracting group experienced more treatment success than the placebo treatment group.

Weathers and Liberman (1975) also used contingency contracting with delinquent boys. Methodological problems make their study difficult to interpret, but generally few positive results were found. It is possible that these adolescents are more disturbed and their families more set in nonproductive patterns of interaction than would be the case with younger hyperactive children.

Contracting has many attributes that make it an attractive intervention technique for use with hyperactive children. Since the parents administer the contract and its consequences, cost in terms of therapist time can be minimized. Moreover, many authors (e.g. Patterson, 1974; Eyberg and Johnson, 1974) have stressed the importance of having parents carry out the behavior modification program in order to maximize generalization and the maintenance of behavior change in the child's natural environment.

During a meeting with Chris' parents, it was decided that the most important behavior to include in an initial contract was tantruming. Both parents were given behavior charts, and asked to record each tantrum without Chris' knowledge. A tantrum was defined as Chris being verbally abusive toward either parent in a loud tone of voice, usually accompanied by crying.

Following a nine-day baseline, a contract was negotiated between Chris and his parents. The first contract was simple, and involved only positive consequences; if Chris had a tantrum-free day, he would be allowed to stay up for an extra half hour beyond his regular bedtime. During this reinforcing event, he could receive the undivided attention of one of his parents, or choose to read or play by himself. In addition, points could be earned for each tantrum-free day, and these points could be accumulated to exchange for a weekend reward. Typical rewards included outings with his parents (something very rewarding to Chris, since both his parents were busy people and his time alone with them was often limited) or small toys or items of sports equipment. Initially, the "cost" of the weekend reward was attainable by Chris with a minimal improvement over baseline. Gradually, following discussion and negotiation with Chris, the number of points required was increased. Details of the initial contract and its subsequent revisions are presented in Table 1.

One week after the contract was in effect, it was altered so that Chris also could earn points toward the weekly reward by clearing his place at the table at all meals, and putting his dirty clothes in the laundry, without argument and with only one prompting from his parents. The extended bedtime remained contingent upon the absence of tantruming behavior during the day, and was not affected by Chris' task completion. Later in the intervention, Chris could earn points for being ready for school on time, being on time for lunch and supper, and doing homework. These behaviors had required constant parental prompting before inclusion in the contract.

Results

In order to assess the effectiveness of contracting, both of Chris' parents completed the Conners' Parent Symptom Questionnaire (Conners, 1970) twice, once before and once after intervention. In addition, they kept recording the frequency of the target behaviors throughout the intervention

TABLE 1

Details of Contingency Contract
Chris B

Behaviors	Days	Points Earned (+) or Lost (—)			
		10-16	17-30	31-58	59-65
		"free" 20			
Doesn't lose temper all day		+5	+5	+5	+5
Loses temper		—5	—5	—5	—5
Clears place at table, 3 meals			+5	+5	+5
			+5	+5	+5
			+5	+5	+5
Clothes put in laundry			+5	+5	+5
Ready for school at 8:00 A.M.				+5	+5
Home for lunch at 12:05 P.M.				+5	+5
Come for supper				+5	+5
Does homework				+5	+5
Maximum number of points possible/week		175	175	315	315
Total points required for reward*		120	120	250	280

* Reward was available each Saturday; it varied from week to week, but was either an outing with parents or a small toy or sports item.

period. They also completed a short questionnaire concerning the effects of contracting.

Behavioral Data. During baseline recording, Chris had an average of 1.44 tantrums/day (see Figure 1). His mother felt that this was an unusually low frequency of tantrums and estimated the typical frequency at five/day. Immediately following institution of the contract (day 10; Figure 1) Chris' frequency of tantrums rose. His parents reported that Chris resisted the contract and told them that if it continued, he would behave "worse than ever." His parents persisted, however, and during the first week, Chris had three tantrum-free days. As the contracting continued, the frequency of Chris' tantruming behavior gradually decreased.

To measure the percentage of reduction in the target behavior, the rate of occurrence for the last nine days was averaged, and subtracted from the nine-day baseline rate. This difference was then divided by the baseline rate. Since Chris had no tantrums during the last nine days of intervention, this resulted in a 100 percent decrease from the baseline rate.

During the first week that points were available for the four tasks, Chris was successful at completing all of them each day. During the next visit, his mother stated that, since Chris was doing so well, he should be able to do his tasks without being prompted. This change was incorporated into the contract and resulted in a decrease in the total number of chores completed during the next six days (see Figure 1, days 24-30). By the following week, Chris was again performing the four tasks without prompting.

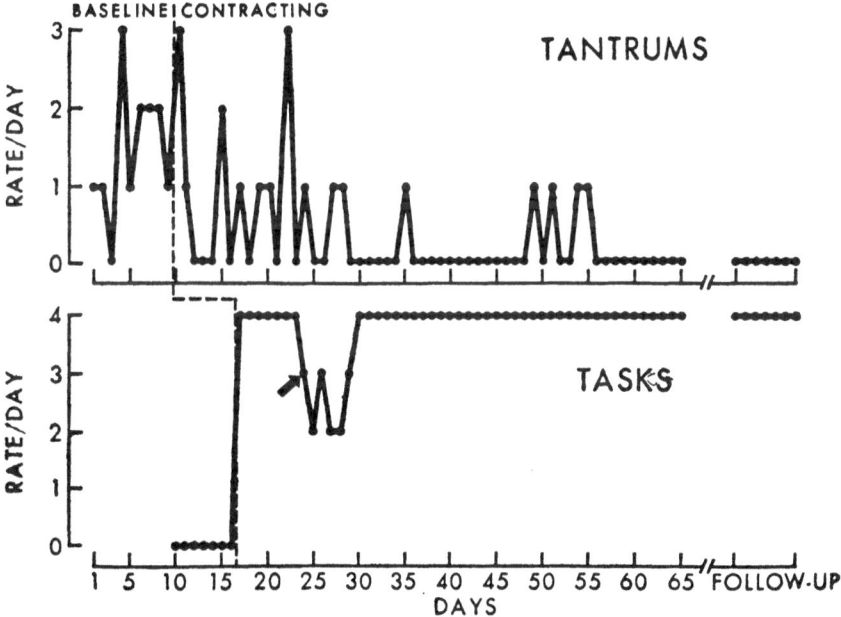

FIG. 1. Chris B. Frequency of tantruming behavior and total daily task completion (possible total of four) recorded by his parents. The arrow at day 20 indicates the point at which promptings for tasks were terminated.

At this time, the therapist suggested to Chris that he begin to monitor his points. Chris subsequently expressed great interest in marking the points on the chart, and added them up each day. This self-charting procedure became an effective reinforcer for Chris' appropriate behaviors. His mother reported that during four different weeks, Chris had accumulated enough points to exchange for his weekend reward by Thursday, but this good behavior was maintained by continuing to record his points on Friday. He became quite competitive with himself, and liked to earn more points each week than he had earned the previous week.

Adding the "being on time" and homework tasks to the contract resulted in an increase in the frequency with which Chris performed those tasks without being disruptive. Although these behaviors were not included in Figure 1, since an adequate baseline was not available, the parents expressed their pleasure in Chris' performance.

Conners' Parent Symptom Questionnaire Data. The mean factor scores of the Conner's Parent Symptom Questionnaires are presented in Table 2. Since each factor consists of a variable number of items, each scored 0 (not at all) to 3 (very much), the total sum for each factor was divided by the number of items to provide a mean score for the factor. Mean scores for the Impulsive-Hyperactive factor decreased .38 (mother) and .25 (father). In addition, mean scores for the Conduct Problem factor were reduced by .85 and .57 for mother and father, respectively. The Learning Problem factor also showed a consistent decrease of .25 and .50, although these scores were not initially very high, even at the time of the pre-test.

TABLE 2

Mean Factor Scores—Conners' Parent Symptom Questionnaire
Chris B

Factor	Mother			Father		
	Pre	Post	Follow-up	Pre	Post	Follow-up
Conduct problem	1.28	.43	.57	1.14	.57	1.00
Anxiety	0	.86	.43	1.14	.71	.43
Impulsive-hyperactive	2.00	1.62	1.62	1.87	1.62	2.00
Learning problem	.25	0	.25	.75	.25	.50
Psychosomatic	0	.20	0	0	.20	0
Perfectionism	2.00	2.00	2.00	2.00	2.30	2.00
Antisocial	0	0	0	0	0	0
Muscular tension	0	0	0	1.25	1.00	.50

Questionnaire Assessment of Contracting. In response to the questionnaire, Chris' mother and father both reported that, as a result of contracting,
Chris' behavior had improved markedly and that they felt much more
positively toward him. They stated that Chris seemed to be happier at
home following intervention, and that their family, on the whole, had begun
to function better as a result of the treatment.

Follow-up

At termination of intervention, Chris' parents were given enough
behavior charts and blank contract forms for several months, and were
not contacted again until three months had passed. At this time, the mother
was contacted by telephone, and asked to record the target behaviors for
a period of one week. In addition, she and her husband completed another
Conners' Parent Symptom Questionnaire. She reported that they were still
using contracting and that Chris remained enthusiastic about the program.

The behavioral data collected during this follow-up indicated that improvement made by the end of intervention had persisted; no tantrums
were recorded by either parent, and Chris was still performing all of his
tasks without without parental reminders. The parents' responses to the
Conners' scale at follow-up are reported in Table 2. Reductions in the
mean scores across the factors were maintained for Chris' mother, while
his father's responses to the Conduct Problem and Impulsive-Hyperactive
factors returned to pre-intervention levels.

Conclusion

Through contingency contracting, this family was able to decrease the
frequency of Chris' tantruming behavior to a level acceptable to them,
within three weeks. In addition, the frequency of appropriate behaviors,
such as the performance of simple household tasks and being punctual
about daily routine, was increased. Positive changes in Chris' behavior
were reflected in his parents' responses to a treatment questionnaire and
the Conners' Parent Symptom Questionnaire. Behavioral improvements
were maintained during a three-month followup. Intervention required
approximately 10 hours and 30 minutes of therapist involvement in home
visits, with an additional 30 minutes spent in telephone contact with the
family. Therefore, a short, time-limited behavioral intervention with contingency contracting was successful in producing positive change in the
behavior of this hyperactive boy, and may be a useful technique for
treatment of hyperactive children on a larger scale.

It should be noted that, in order to be successful, the contract must be simple enough for the child to understand, and be kept as positive as possible. The therapist and parents often will require ingenuity in determining suitable reinforcers and, in addition, must keep the contracting procedure flexible enough to adapt to the changing needs of the family.

References

CONNERS, C. K. Symptom patterns in hyperkinetic, neurotic, and normal children. *Child Dev.* 1970, 41:667-682.

EYBERG, S. M. and JOHNSON, S. M. Multiple assessment of behavior modification with families: Effects of contingency contracting and order of treated problems. *J. Consulting and Clin. Psychol.* 1974, 42:594-606.

HOMME, L., CSANYI, A. P., GONZALES, M. A., and RECHS, J. R. *How to Use Contingency Contracting in the Classroom.* Champaign, Ill.: Research Press, 1969.

PATTERSON, G. R. Interventions with boys with conduct problems: Multiple settings, treatments and criteria. *J. Consulting and Clin. Psychol.* 1974, 42:471-482.

STUART, R. B. Behavioral contracting within families of delinquents. *J. Behav. Ther. and Exp. Psychiat.* 1971, 2:1-11.

STUART, R. B., JAYARATNE, S., and TRIPOLDI, T. Changing adolescent deviant behavior through reprogramming the behavior of parents and teachers: An experimental evaluation. *Canadian J. Behav. Sci.* 1976, 8:132-143.

WEATHERS, L. and LIBERMAN, R. P. Contingency contracting with families of delinquent adolescents. *Behav. Ther.* 1975, 6:356-366.

CHAPTER 3

Autogenic Training:
Learning Body Control

An early notion regarding the hyperactive child had to do with "driven" behavior. The child seemed to lack appropriate inhibitory capabilities, hypothetically due to quirks of development or to some central nervous system trauma, and, consequently, the child reacted impulsively to stimuli.

The presumed involuntary nature of the behavior and the belief that the child was incapable of self-management, invited interventions that were external to the child. Medication, for example, was not used to "cure" the condition but, rather, to reduce the deleterious symptoms of hyperactivity until the child "outgrew" it. The environmental destimulation model was also based on the beliefs that the child was incapable of managing his attentional processes and, therefore, needed to be in a special learning environment.

The hope offered by such autogenic procedures as biofeedback and systematic relaxation training, is to increase the child's capacity for self-management. The potential for individuals to control autonomic functions, formerly considered beyond conscious control, is only now being tapped (Green, 1977; Brown, 1974). The focus of this chapter will be specific to hyperactive children.

A review of the literature revealed a variety of self-management programs. There are reports of muscle-relaxation training (Braud et al., 1975;

Jeffrey, 1976) temperature training (Martin and Hersey, 1976), alpha training (Nall, 1973) and systematic relaxation training (Klein, 1977; Lupin et al., 1976).

Some of the reported programs used several procedures concomitantly. For example, Simpson and Nelson (1974) used reinforcement procedures along with breathing-pattern feedback to assist a group of hyperactive children in modifying their behavior. Jeffery (1976) also used operant conditioning procedures along with an electromyographic (muscle control) program.

The published literature has generally been positive in demonstrating that hyperactive children are capable of increased self-management. Carry-over from training sessions into the classroom and home have been reported. The several studies being presented in this chapter cover a range of procedures and also illustrate how different procedures can be effectively combined.

References

BRAUD, L. W., LUPIN, M. N., and BRAUD, W. G. The use of electromyographic biofeedback in the control of hyperactivity. *J. Learning Dis.* 1975, 8:420-425.

BROWN, B. B. *New Mind, New Body.* New York: Harper & Row, 1974.

GREEN, E. and A. *Beyond Biofeedback.* New York: Dell Publishing Co., 1977.

JEFFERY, T. B. The effects of operant conditioning and electromyographic biofeedback on the relaxed behavior of hyperkinetic children. *Dissertation Abstracts.* 1976, 37:2510.

KLEIN, S. A. Relaxation and exercise for hyperactive, impulsive children. *Dissertation Abstracts.* 1977, 37:6334.

LUPIN, M., BRAUD, L. B., BRAUD, W., and DUER, W. F. Children, parents and relaxation tapes. *Acad. Ther.* 1976, 12:105-113.

MARTIN, L. L. and HERSEY, M. An exploratory investigation of the effect of a biofeedback technique with hyperactive, learning disabled children. Paper presented at the International Convention of the Counsel for Exceptional Children, Chicago, April 4-9, 1976.

NALL, A. Alpha training and the hyperactive child . . . is it effective? *Acad. Ther.* 1973, 9:5-19.

SIMPSON, D. D. and NELSON, A. E. Attention training through breathing control to modify hyperactivity. *J. Learning Dis.* 1974, 7:274-283.

CASE STUDY #7. THE EFFECTS OF BIOFEEDBACK TRAINING ON AN EIGHT-YEAR-OLD BOY

Vivien J. Worster

Current Problem

Richard is an eight-year-old who was recommended for biofeedback training because of his difficulty in concentrating on his work, his inability to finish his classwork, and his disruptive behavior in class. His teacher had verbally reprimanded him, taken away privileges in class, and used corporal punishment as a means to control his behavior and get him to complete his work. Limited success was reported with these approaches. Comments by the teacher describing Richard's performance and behavior included, "I know he can do the work; he just won't concentrate; he is fidgety, he is out to show-off, he seldom completes assignments, he rarely follows direction, and he does not attempt difficult tasks."

On the playground and in the community, Richard was antagonistic toward peers and had poor relationships with them. The teacher reports that he is sometimes withdrawn. His mother reports satisfactory adjustment at home and in the community.

Background Information

The following information was obtained by the school psychologist in a parent interview and through testing. Richard was born one month premature, remaining in the hospital for seven days. He was reported to have had many colds during his first year of life. Richard is an only child, and his parents were divorced when Richard was six-years old. When Richard was seven, his mother remarried. Richard reported that he does not interact with his stepfather very much, mainly because of his stepfather working the 4:00 p.m. to 12:00 a.m. shift at a local factory. Richard's mother reported that her son has few responsibilities at home. According to her, he likes to play very much, but is disinterested in games that have much structure or many rules. Richard antagonizes friends while playing with them and displays difficulty handling peer relationships.

Discipline at home was characterized as being easy and lenient. Methods for disciplining included grounding, restriction to the yard, limiting bike riding, and a few spankings. Richard repeated the first grade due primarily to his inability to complete assigned work.

The WISC-R, Peabody Picture Vocabulary Test, Bender-Gestalt, and the Wide Range Achievement Test were administered in the second month of the third grade. Richard's full-scale I.Q. was reported as falling within the normal range, with his PPVT I.Q. falling in the superior range. The school psychologist reported results of the Bender-Gestalt reflected Richard's observable behavior as reported by school personnel. Also noted was difficulty in handling fear-producing interpersonal relationships, anxiety and self-doubt, inability to complete tasks, impaired reality testing, and possible organicity. Administration of the WISC-R revealed distractibility, anxiety, possible organic impairment, lack of concentration, and frustration.

Intervention

Intervention consisted of biofeedback training using a thermal trainer and electromyograph. The target area concentrated on was "increasing Richard's self-concept." Measures of this were obtained by administering the Sears Self Concept Rating Scale before the first session and after the twelfth session. Teacher ratings of Richard's behavior were obtained before and after intervention, using the Four Quay Dimensions of Behavior Disorders as well as a report from the parents (mother responded on questionnaire).

It appeared that Richard's parent-child relationship had tolerated and possibly reinforced his pattern of behavior. The assumption of the intervention strategy was that Richard's self-concept would improve through biofeedback training and also that his concentration and self-control would improve as measured by the Sears Scale and teacher and parent reports.

Richard was seen by a therapist every Tuesday and Thursday for half an hour over a six-week period. Biofeedback training consisted of six half-hour sessions using the thermal trainer and six half-hour sessions using the electromyograph. A record of beginning and ending finger temperature was taken, as well as beginning and ending microvolt outputs of the frontalis muscle group. Richard made steady improvement and gained mastery over controlling his external skin temperature and reducing muscle activity.

Conclusion

Richard demonstrated improved control over his physical processes of external skin temperature and reduced muscle activity. His self-concept improved significantly, according to comparison of pre- and post-treatment scores on the Sears Self Concept Scale (pretest score: 3.16; post-test score: 3.77).

The teacher reported a dramatic improvement in Richard; he began completing his work and was observed to be concentrating more intently and for longer periods of time than had been previously noted. Richard's mother noted on the post-treatment interview that there was marked improvement in his physical self-control and school attendance, and a marked decrease in shyness.

CASE STUDY #8. THE USE OF BIOFEEDBACK TRAINING ON A NINE-YEAR-OLD CHILD

Vivien J. Worster

Current Problem

The student, Karen, is nine years old and is enrolled in the second grade. She was referred by her teacher for biofeedback training due to her exhibiting the following behaviors in the classroom: attention seeking (getting out of her seat often); failure to complete work; playing with toys during classtime; hypersensitivity; lack of self-confidence; and fear and anxiousness. Karen's mother used the term "hyperactive" when describing her daughter's behavior and remarked that she seemed "flighty," overly sensitive, and had difficulty concentrating or remaining still. Karen often complained of being unable to sleep at night and expressed much anxiety about an upcoming stay in the hospital for a tonsilectomy. She attended special reading classes and was relatively behind other same-aged students in academic achievement. Her teacher perceived her problems in school as due to "emotional insecurities" and recommended her for treatment, feeling that Karen would benefit from biofeedback training.

Background Information

Karen is the fourth of five siblings. She resides with her mother, stepfather, and one younger brother. Karen's natural father left the family when she was three years old. He lives in a nearby town with the three eldest siblings, but refuses to visit Karen. The mother has told her that her father is "far away" in order to spare her feelings, but Karen continues to ask about her absent father.

When Karen was one year old, her mother became pregnant with a female child who died shorlty after birth. Although the mother states that Karen was too young to remember her sister, she states that she herself was extremely depressed over the child's death and mourned for a lengthy time, keeping pictures of the dead child in view around the home.

Following the pregnancy with her sixth child, the mother developed a cancerous tumor and was hospitalized for two months. During this time, Karen was left in the charge of a series of baby-sitters. An elderly baby-sitter who stayed with her, and of whom she was quite fond, died when Karen was four. Karen's mother states that Karen was very unhappy at this time and feared her mother would not return from the hospital. After the mother's recovery, she remarried and began working. She remembers this as a difficult time, as Karen cried each time she left for work.

Karen entered kindergarten at the age of six. At this time, Karen's mother noted that Karen became very emotional and cried each day upon returning from school. Karen was taken to a clinic for testing and consultation. The testing revealed a normal I.Q. and no evidence of organic complications. Karen was kept out of kindergarten for that year and seemed more favorably adjusted when she returned to school. Karen's mother expressed concern over the child's extreme sensitivity, lack of concentration, and "flightiness." Karen's difficulty sleeping and repeated questioning about her father's absence are also of concern to her mother.

Intervention

Karen is currently receiving biofeedback training with the thermal trainer and electromyograph. She has completed six sessions of thermal training and three sessions of electromyograph training. The sessions total 45 minutes in length with 30 minutes spent in actual training and 15 minutes devoted to reviewing the session or playing structured games.

The thermal training was conducted as follows: After the sensor was attached to the forefinger and a baseline reading taken, Karen was instructed to sit quietly and imagine warmth flowing from the top of her head through her neck, shoulders, and finally into the tips of her fingers. Deep breathing and relaxation exercises were also utilized, and the student was instructed to pay special attention to how her body felt in this relaxed state. In the initial three sessions Karen raised her digital temperature an average of four degrees. By the fourth session, she increased to 90 degrees from a baseline of 82 degrees. She demonstrated this ability equally well on both hands. Feedback and reinforcement for each increase consisted of light, sound, and verbal praise from the therapist.

Training with the EMG was conducted in basically the same manner, except that Karen was instructed to experience looseness and relaxation across the frontalis muscle, neck, and shoulders. She began training at a level of six 1-100 microvolts and is presently working successfully at a setting of three and a half 1-100 microvolts. To vary the training procedure and insure retention of thermal training, Karen has worked with both instruments simultaneously. She is instructed to raise her temperature and keep the sound to a minimum on the EMG. She is able to perform both operations with an increasing degree of success.

During the training sessions, Karen has spoken to the therapist about her difficulty sleeping. It has been suggested that she practice relaxation before going to bed. In a conference with her mother, it was suggested that she also practice relaxation exercises with Karen, using thermal strips for home practice.

Karen has also expressed sadness and confusion concerning her sister's death and her father's absence during the sessions. At one point in a latter part of the session, she drew a hospital and transformed it into a "monster's house," where the nurse becomes a witch with evil intentions. In discussing the picture with Karen, it would appear that her fear of the hospital is largely due to the history of illness, death, and separation in her family.

Conclusion

Although the treatment is not completed at the time of this writing, Karen appears to have improved in several areas as the training has progressed. Her teacher has remarked that she gets out of her seat less often, completes more assigned work, and has begun developing friendships with other students in the class. During an interview, Karen's mother also commented that Karen seemed "more relaxed and less flighty." The mother recalled one occasion recently when Karen had to wait in the car for her stepfather. She remarked that Karen sat quietly and read a book. Prior to treatment, the mother recalls that it was very difficult for Karen to sit still in the car and remarked that she would change positions rapidly and appear agitated.

The therapist has further observed that Karen appears less anxious and displays greater ability to concentrate now than in earlier sessions. She exhibits less fidgeting during sessions and appears to attend more to the therapist and instruments with less idle glancing around the room. Karen has responded enthusiastically to the training and seems pleased with her success. Speaking of the training, she remarked, "I sleep better now and it's easier to get my work done." It would appear that the previous unstable family situation, separation from her mother, and confusion regarding her father's whereabouts may have produced in Karen much anxiety and insecurity. The biofeedback training, with its focus on relaxation and body awareness, coupled with the positive feelings she received from success with the instruments, may account for the positive behavioral changes.

CASE STUDY #9. RELAXATION THERAPY WITH A HYPERACTIVE SIX-YEAR-OLD CHILD

Mimi Lupin

Current Problem

Johnny was an extremely hyperactive six-year-old child. He was having a great deal of difficulty in school, even though he was repeating kindergarten. He was unable to perform simple fine motor tasks, and his extremely hyperactive behavior was distracting to both the teacher and other students. Johnny was unable to attend to an assigned task for longer than a second or two before he was off on his own, playing with something else or wandering around the room. The teacher also commented that his peer relations were poor; he teased and hit other children and whined to get his way. The teacher felt that even though he was six and a half, he was not ready for the first grade.

Background Information

When Johnny was two and a half years old, he was in a auto accident that left him with a ruptured spleen, collapsed lung, and a severe brain concussion. As he grew older, he became noticeably hyperactive, and it appeared that he was getting progressively worse. His mother had taken him to a number of doctors for help, but none was forthcoming. His pediatrician prescribed medication to help him relax enough to fall asleep. Several drugs were tried before the combination of 100 mg of Deaner, an older but lesser known drug, and 100 mg of Thorazine proved to be somewhat effective. As a result, his sleeping problems diminished and his attention span improved somewhat. However his mother became increasingly concerned about the possible effect of the drugs upon Johnny's height and weight. He looked more like a four-year-old child than one who was six and a half.

During his second year in kindergarten, he was tested with the Wechsler Intelligence Scale for Children and the following Scores were obtained: a Verbal I.Q. Score of 74; a Performance I.Q. Score of 60; and a Full Scale I.Q. Score of 64. Several physicians had suggested to Johnny's mother that she place him in a residential treatment center on the basis of his behavior and test scores. She maintained that, although his test scores indicated so, she felt that he was not mentally retarded. She did acknowledge his extreme difficulty in relating to other children, and found his aggressive behavior very disruptive to the entire family. She also said that he had frequent temper tantrums that lasted for 35 to 40 minutes and that the least little thing prompted them. It had gotten to the point that she was unable to even take him to the grocery store. His mother commented hat she was "at the end of her rope," and when the school psychologist suggested the use of a relaxation program that could be used at home, the mother was very receptive.

Intervention

The school psychologist developed a series of relaxation exercises and stories patterned after Jacobson's relaxation exercises (Lupin, 1977b). To avoid boredom with the exercises, the stories were developed to incorporate a shortened version of the exercises as well as soothing sounds (i.e., ocean waves, music, sounds of birds, brooks, etc.) and they offered more appropriate ways to deal with situations that children face in their daily lives. As these ideas were offered within a story line, Kenny was more able to accept the suggested behaviors without contest.

The psychologist recommended that Kenny use the relaxation tape daily before bedtime for three weeks, after which he would use the story tapes in the suggested sequential order. After using the story tapes in sequence for three times, Johnny was allowed to choose his favorite story to play nightly thereafter. Every third or fourth night, he used the basic relaxation tape before listening to his story tape. Kenny's mother supervised the use of the tapes during the first three weeks and thereafter only when he used the relaxation tape. She followed instructions similar to the ones given below:

First, find a comfortable place to lie down. You may use a small pillow if you choose. Loosen any tight clothing. You may wish to remove your shoes.

(1) To begin, close your eyes as tightly as you can. Hold for the count of five. Then, relax the eyes, letting go all the tension in the eyes. Take a deep breath, and let it go slowly.

(2) Raise your eyebrows up as high as you can. Hold for the count of five. Then let go all the tension.

(3) Open your mouth as wide as possible and hold for the count of five. Relax and let go.

(4) Stick out your tongue as far as possible and feel the tension in your neck. Hold for the count of five. Relax and let go. Take a deep breath and let it out slowly.

(5) Now, raise your shoulders up under your ears and hold them as tightly as possible. Feel the tension in your shoulders. Hold for the count of five and let go.

(6) Now, make a fist with both hands. Hold them as tightly as possible for the count of five, then relax them and let go all tension in the arms and hands.

(7) Next, pull in your stomach as though you were trying to touch your stomach to your backbone. Feel the tension in your stomach. Hold it to the count of five. Relax and let go all the tension in your stomach. Take a deep breath and let it go slowly.

(8) As tightly as possible, squeeze your buttocks together and hold for the count of five. Feel the tension in your buttocks and upper legs. Take a deep breath and let go all the tension slowly. Feel the warm feelings of relaxation spreading into your buttocks and upper legs.

(9) Press your heels into the floor as hard as you can, pulling your toes toward your face. Feel the tension in the backs of your legs. Hold for the count of five, and then relax and let go all the tension. See how good it feels to release all the tension. Take a deep breath and let it go slowly. As you breathe out, feel all the tension leaving your body.

(10) Now press your heels into the floor and point your toes away from your face. Feel the tension in the tops of your legs and ankles. Hold for the count of five. Then let go and relax completely. Now that you have experienced how it feels to be very tense, and very relaxed, you will soon become aware of when your muscles feel tight and be able to relax by taking a deep breath and letting go all the tension.

By taking a deep breath and relaxing when you are angry or afraid, you will be able to handle the situation better. It is important to let all body parts stay relaxed while tensing only one part. This may be difficult at first, but as you practice, it will become easier.

Before the beginning of each session, Johnny removed his shoes and loosened his clothing. At first he refused to cooperate, but his mother allowed him to complete only a couple of minutes of the exercise each time and offered him a treat as an incentive. Each time, he was required to complete a little more of the tape to get his reward. Later, Johnny began to fall asleep by the end of the tape and the rewards were discontinued. As he began to feel better as the result of relaxation training, he was no longer opposed to using the tape.

His mother also discussed Johnny's treatment plan with his teacher. She was asked to quietly remind Johnny to relax when he became upset or hyperactive or when he began to have difficulty with his peers. The teacher reported that when such an incident occurred, she would find a puzzle or game for Johnny to become involved in, so that he could spend a few minutes alone to become relaxed again. She also encouraged him to verbalize his anger appropriately which further reduced his tension.

After Johnny had used the basic tape for about three weeks, his mother began to reduce his level of medication gradually over the next three-week period. Six weeks after he began using the tapes, he was no longer on medication and went to sleep within 10 to 15 minutes after going to bed, often during his story tape. Previously, it had taken him one and a half to two hours to fall asleep.

Conclusion

Three months after Johnny's treatment began, a very definite improvement could be observed. He no longer looked at though he were drugged, and he was physically alert. He was less quarrelsome and got along better with peers. Although he was still somewhat hyperactive, he had improved dramatically, considering the severity of his problem. His mother reported that even the neighbors who knew nothing of Johnny's treatment commented on how well he was playing with the other children on the block. She said that he would go for three or four days without a squabble, whereas previously he was fighting almost constantly. As a result of his improved friendships and self control, Johnny's teacher and parents noted an improvement in his self esteem as well. Before, his favorite words had been "I can't," and this was said in a whiny voice. After treatment, he would comment, "I'm doing better aren't I?" or "Look what I did!" He was praised for his accomplishments by both teacher and parents. His teacher reported an increase in Johnny's attention span, although it still was not as good as that of the other class members.

Johnny was tested shortly after the three-month period by a school psychologist who had no knowledge of his treatment. Testing was done in order to meet state requirements for entrance to special classes for the mentally retarded. No remediation was given between pre- and post-testing sessions. The WISC test scores were as follows: Verbal I.Q. Score of 99 (an increase of 25 points); a Performance I.Q. Score of 65 (an increase of 5 points); and a Full Scale I.Q. Score of 81 (an increase of 17 points). His mother was extremely pleased with his test scores as she always maintained that he was not mentally retarded.

As can be seen by the comparison of the pretest and post-test, Johnny was found not mentally retarded, as his mother had always maintained. He was considered to be a minimal brain injured (M.B.I.) child, with depressed scores due to his previous inability to attend to the testing session long enough for an accurate diagnosis to be made. After post-testing, it became apparent that he had great deficits in the performance skills areas due to brain injury, and verbal scores were depressed due to his inability to attend. His M.B.I. pattern was "masked" due to the depression of his verbal scores. After the post-testing was completed, the school began an intensive remediation program in fine motor skills. It was also emphasized that he continue relaxation training, as relaxation training has been shown to improve fine motor skills (Braud, 1978; Carter, 1974).

Since the post-test Johnny's family has moved out of town, and there has not been further testing after his remediation. With the improvement in his fine motor skills, Johnny's teacher felt that a retest would show further improvement in his performance skills on the WISC, which would reflect on the total I.Q. score. Although after several months of treatment Johnny was still more active than the normal child, he had come a long way in controlling his aggression and in the development of better self esteem.

Relaxation, of course, is not a panacea for the hyperactive child. It has been observed, however, that relaxation does tend to reduce aggressive behavior and does help the child develop self-control, which seems to have advantages over the use of medication.

References

BRAUD, L. W. The effects of EMG biofeedback and progressive relaxation upon hyperactivity and its behavioral concommitants. *J. of Biofeedback*. 1978, in press.

CARTER, J. and SYNOLDS, D. Effects of relaxation training upon handwriting quality. *J. Learning Dis.* 1974, 7:236-238.

LUPIN, M. *Peace, Harmony Awareness: A Family Relaxation Program.* Houston, Texas: Self Management Tapes, 1977. (a)

LUPIN, M. *Peace, Harmony Awareness: A Relaxation Program for Children.* Austin, Texas: Learning Concepts, 1977. (b)

CASE STUDY #10. THE ECLECTIC USE OF BIOFEEDBACK, BEHAVIOR THERAPY AND THERAPEUTIC COUNSELING BY A MALE/FEMALE TEAM IN EFFECTIVELY TREATING HYPERKINESIS

Norma Estrada

Current Problem

Corey, a seven-year-old was brought by his parents for consultation because of his excessive physical activity, short attention span, and the resulting school problems due to his erratic behavior. When Corey came for treatment, he was on a drug regimen of Ritalin, 10 mg., taken two to three times a day. He was not sleeping well and had a poor appetite. His parents described him as a "textbook case of MBD," although there were no records of impairment or organic brain dysfunction. Corey's parents were concerned about the use of drugs and were seeking an alternative to drug therapy. A family friend had suggested biofeedback.

In school, Corey could not sit still and was not completing his homework assignments. There was some recent academic improvement because of his admiration for his current teacher, who was supportive and positive in her praise of his achievements. He was having problems in arithmetic and his lack of interest in the reading material interfered with his reading scores. On testing, just prior to our consultation, special attention was focused on Corey's choice of eye dominance. He seemed to be left-handed for most fine-motor tasks, yet chose his right hand for throwing. He showed difficulty with gross motor tasks as well as fine motor skills. The results of testing also showed the areas of dysfunction to be in number reversals, regrouping in addition, fine-motor coordination, motor planning, and organizational skills. He was easily distracted and did not follow directions. He was, however, accepted as a third-grade student, needing supplemental assistance from a resource or learning teacher.

His inability to relate to his peers at school led to social isolation during lunch and recreation periods. In his home community, his ineffective behavior with children his own age prevailed, and he would seek out children younger than himself to play with. He would often take advantage of them, however, and because of this abuse, was forbidden to play with anyone younger than himself. As a result, he was spending his time alone at home watching television. He seemed preoccupied with the acquisition of money and on his excursions away from home would check coin slots in any establishment he happened to be in. During one such episode, his hand became firmly lodged in a coin slot and had to be removed with assistance from the fire department.

Background Information

The following background information was obtained from Corey's parents. Corey was a full-term baby and pregnancy was uneventful. There are no siblings. With the exception of pneumonia, there had been no other significant illnesses. His first three developmental years were normal.

His father, a successful businessman, was away from home except for weekends until Corey was three years old. During this period, his mother relates a happy, close relationship with Corey with no noticeable behavioral or health problems. He was considered to be bright, active, and alert.

When Corey was three years of age, his father resumed full residence in their home. It was at about this time that Corey's behavior began to change. The family moved to their present location when Corey was approximately four years of age. Prior to the move, the pediatrician had placed him on Ritalin. The real difficulties began when Corey entered school. He was disruptive, had a short attention span, and, although he was considered to be bright, his behavior was interfering with his progress in school.

The qualities of hyperactivity had been described as being present in the behavior pattern of both the father and his family. All the members of the family are dynamic, creative, active, and successful in their chosen professions, including Corey's 73-year-old grandmother. They abound with energy and initiative that appears to be above the accepted norm. Corey's mother considers herself to have the same qualities to a lesser degree.

Intervention

The eclectic model use for intervention included biofeedback, behavior therapy, and therapeutic counseling by a male/female team.

The biofeedback sessions were designed to enable Corey to play a more important part in controlling his own behavior and were focused on providing physiologic information about the ways in which he could achieve a mastery of his own internal functioning. Research studies demonstrate that a systematic approach for the learning of internal awareness and control promotes creativity and improved communication skills, as well as a reduction in somatic symptomatology (Englehardt, 1976; Haight et al., 1976; King, 1972).

Corey was first taught to warm his hands. Hand-warming is done with relative ease by children and is a tangible indication of progress. It requires quieting the autonomic nervous system and is a reflection of increased blood supply to the peripheral vessels of the hand. The training sessions consisted of attaching a sensitive thermister to the index finger of Corey's dominant hand. As Corey became adept at hand-warming, the thermister was moved from one hand to the other. At his request, the thermister was moved to his feet which he soon learned to warm just as easily as his hands. The instrument used was a large dial thermometer with visual and audio feedback.

By learning to control muscle activity in the frontalis and trapezias muscles with the use of an electromyograph, Corey was able to sit quietly for longer periods of time, thus eliminating his restless behavior. The electromyograph picked up activity at the myoneural junction and monitored muscle activity. Feedback was both visual and audio. Research suggesting that the ability to inhibit motor movement improves cognitive performance (Maccoby ct al., 1965), and, more recently, the report by Lubar and Shouse (1976) on the use of biofeedback EEG to teach control of the sensorimotor rhythm in children in order to enhance motor inhibition, since the rhythm's most characteristic behavioral correlate is immobility, influenced our exploration of the learned control of excess activity in striate muscles.

When Corey had mastered hand-warming and muscle control, we introduced brain-wave training. Our baseline statistics and EEG readings on the five hyperkinetic children we have worked with have shown a predominance of alpha waves (sub-beta). Most therapeutic and experiential descriptions of sub-beta mental states are characterized as being relaxed and pleasant. Some individuls, however, involuntarily, habitually, or spasmodically become "fixed" in these states. Recent research has demonstrated that these fixed states can be both unpleasant and impairing (Mikuriya et al., 1977).

Psychophysiological factors influencing EEG activity are the primary emphasis of researchers and clinicians involved in biofeedback encephalography (*Handbook of Physiologic Feedback*, Vol. 1, 1976). According to classical thinking, there are four primary EEG rhythms, which are classified according to their dominant frequency. Each of these frequency bands is correlated with a general mental arousal level and associated with a set of generalized behavioral correlates. *Beta* rhythm (above 13 Hz.) is characterized by active concentration, directed attention to external arousal. *Alpha* rhythm (8-13 Hz.) is characterized by slow waves, and is considered to be a relief from focused attention and certain forms of cognitive activity, a low mental arousal level, and passive attention to external stimuli. *Theta* rhythm (4-8 Hz.) is characterized by drowsiness, dreaming, hypnogogic imagery, and a lower arousal level than is characterized by alpha rhythm. *Delta* rhythm (0.5-4 Hz.) is characterized by deep, dreamless sleep, it is lowest mental arousal level.

Corey's baseline EEG readings showed a "fixed" alpha-theta state. Beta brain-wave training was introduced in order to enable him to focus his attention for longer periods of time. As focused attention increased, learning impairment decreased. Brain-wave training sessions consisted of placing simple sponge electrodes over the area of the skull responding to the dominant visual cortex. Corey then learned to produce predominant beta waves (fast waves, above 13 Hz.) for periods of up to 20 minutes per session. Since the child could see and hear his brain waves function, he learned to differentiate and identify the subjective correlates representing the state. The ability to focus at will was thus developed.

Adjunctive intervention consisted of introducing fine motor tasks, as well as gross motor skills, into the training sessions. Paper and pencil tasks and puzzles were introduced while Corey was still on the instruments to reinforce eye/hand coordination. Motor reinforcement consisted of exposure to upper-extremity coordination skills, visual perceptual development, awareness of body image and control, and basic reinforcement of self-esteem. Gross motor skills were introduced as homework assignments. These included simple tasks that covered coordination; balance; flexibility; etc., such as throwing a ball against a target.

Behavior therapy followed a modified contingency management model, and was introduced into the training sessions as Corey became more adept at internal control. We worked with Corey on developing more appropriate behavior in his social interaction with his peers. With the female therapist as a model "friend," a hypothetical lunch period was "played out" in verbal conversation while Corey could "see" his physiologic response on the instruments. Appropriate adjustments were made both in the response and the behavior during these sessions, and when satisfaction was achieved by both the child and the therapist, the transfer of the learned behavior from the "therapeutic" to the "natural" setting was attempted. By the end of the tenth visit, Corey very happily reported on his "real" friend. At termination of treatment, his parents reported on his first real relationship with his new friend, Tom. This was the most important reward Corey had received in a long time.

Supportive counseling with the parents took place throughout the training sessions. Periodic progress sessions with parents, therapists, and child were usually short in duration. Emphasis was placed on a relaxed, non-threatening atmosphere with all members participating for effective change, using simplistic and practical methods for systematic integration of the new "learned" behavior. As Corey's behavior began to change, relationships within the family constellation also changed, resulting in the need for parental counseling and supportive, positive suggestions for implementation of healthier physical and social attitudes.

The male/female team provides a comfortable emotional climate and is easily identified by the child, in that it mirrors his own family constellation. It offers the therapists an opportunity for modeling, both for parents and child, and facilitates learning. This approach appears to be particularly helpful to children and allows the freedom of shifting relationships in order to bring about change for child and therapist, eliminating dependency and promoting healthy male/female attitudes. The underlying premise is to move the child from an external locus of control to an internal one. Self-regulation is viewed as a basic shift of responsibility back to the child, resulting in a psychophysiologic "freeing" effect that allows him to increase his relative responses. An increase in self-esteem is one desirable result.

Conclusion

Treatment was terminated on the 16th visit. At the time of termination, Corey had been free of drug therapy for five months. His school report showed excellent progress in arithmetic and reading. His teacher described his behavior in class as being likeable and friendly. He had also established a firm relationship with two new friends his own age. His parents described a better sleeping pattern and a healthier appetite, as well as a more manageable child.

A one year follow-up interview showed Corey completely free of medication, doing above average in his schoolwork, and well-liked by both peers and elders. When asked if he still practiced his internal controls, he answered, "I don't have to because I'm not nervous anymore, I'm just relaxed."

Although this is a very complex therapeutic model, seven-year-olds have little difficulty implementing the learning when it is presented in a simple manner. The sense of mastery achieved from the knowledge of the learned control is pervasive and tends to spread to all areas of the child's functioning.

The rationale for this treatment model proposes that: 1) Quieting the autonomic nervous system has a pervasive effect which includes normalization of homeostatic balance; 2) Inhibition of motor activity in striate muscle by internal control prepares and facilitates perception; 3) Identification and control of brain-wave activity leads to subjective correlates that allow selective attention states and contribute to the development of healthier "cognitive style"; and 4) The sense of mastery gained from the learned control transfers to external, subjective behavior correlates that improve the quality of life.

References

ENGLEHARDT, L. J. The application of biofeedback techniques within a public school setting. Paper presented at the Biofeedback Research Society, Seventh Annual Meeting, Colorado Springs, Colorado, March 1, 1976.

HAIGHT, M. D., IRVINE, A. G., and JAMPOLSKY, G. B. Response of hyperkinesis to EMG biofeedback. Paper presented at Biofeedback Research Society, Seventh Annual Meeting, Colorado Springs, Colorado, March 1, 1976.

Handbook of Physiologic Feedback (Vol 1). Berkeley, Calif.: Autogenics Systems, Inc., 1976.

KING, M. Individualized instruction in continuation high school: Brainwave biofeedback as a science lesson. Paper presented at First Western Area Convention, National Science Teacher Association, San Diego, California, December 2, 1972.

LUBAR, J. F. and SHOUSE, M. N. EEG and behavioral changes in a hyperkinetic child concurrent with training of the sensorimotor rhythm (SMR): A preliminary report. *Biofeedback and Self-regulation.* 1976, 3:293-306.

MACCOBY, E. E., DOWLEY, E. M., HAGEN, J. W., and DEGERMAN, R. Activity level and intellectual functioning in normal preschool children. *Child Dev.* 1965, 36: 761-770.

MIKURIYA, T. D., PELLETIER, K. R., and GLADMAN, A. E. Spasmodic acute and chronic dysrhythmic sub-beta EEG: Psychiatric implications. Paper presented at the Third Annual Meeting, Biofeedback Society of California, Claremont, California, November 11, 1977.

HEWETT, F. Educational programs for children with behavior disorders. In Quay, H. and Werry, J. (eds.), *Psychopathological Disorders of Childhood.* New York: Wiley, 1972.

KEOGH, B. Hyperactivity and learning disorders: Review and speculation. *Except. Child.* 1971, 38:101-109.

CHAPTER 4

Psychoeducational
Intervention

Hyperactive children not only present behavioral problems at home and in school, but very importantly often experience learning problems. By the time hyperactive children have completed elementary school, 70 percent have failed in one grade, and, as a group, they receive lower grades than their non-hyperactive counterparts (Douglas, 1972).

Attempts to understand and explain the learning and performance difficulties of hyperactive children have considered different theories and conjecture. Keogh (1971) identified three main hypotheses: (a) neurological impairment; (b) interference with the acquisition of information because of attention deficits; and (c) faulty decision making due to impulsivity. Each of these hypotheses leads to different intervention strategies. Dyck (1977), in her review of the literature on hyperactivity and learning concluded,

> Hyperactive children, regardless of the etiology of the problem, appear to profit from highly structured environments, time, activities, rewards, and tasks. Although there are variations of the theme of structure, the concept appears with persistence and forms the primary basis for educational management of hyperactive children (p. 118).

Psychoeducational intervention is concerned with the children's learning and academic performance, as much as with the social and personal adjustment aspects of the hyperactive pattern. Typically, the focus of intervention is on increasing academic attainment. The hyperactive pattern (distractability, fidgetiness, excess movements, etc.) is considered in relation to its interaction with the learning process.

The literature has identified four important considerations related to psychoeducational intervention:

(a) *The stimulus characteristics of the environment.* The position espoused by Cruikshank and his coworkers (Cruikshank et al., 1961) is still popular, in terms of the hyperactive child being unable to adequately process multiple stimuli. From this view, care needs to be exercised in the monitoring of auditory and visual stimuli. This involves considerations of where the child is seated, the selective use of cubicles or partitions, and the stimulus value of the material to be learned.

(b) *The structure of reinforcement.* Some children will work for a future reward, while other children seem unable to delay gratification and, instead, require more immediate reinforcement. The latter seems to be the case with many hyperactive children. Freibergs and Douglas (1969) reported a study wherein hyperactive children were able to perform as well as normal children on concept-learning tasks under the condition of continuous reinforcement. Under only partial reinforcement, however, the quality of performance decreased for the hyperactive children.

(c) *The sequencing of experiences.* For many hyperactive children, the curricular experiences are incongruent with their skill level, readiness to attend, capacity to deal with long-term tasks, and ability to work independently. Hewett (1972), in particular, has addressed himself to the importance of engineering the environment so that it matches where the child is, in terms of his readiness to learn. Tasks are organized and presented so as to increase the likelihood of success. There is extensive structuring of the tasks and expectations, coupled with relatively immediate feedback, so as to accommodate the child's readiness to perform. As the child's self-directedness and readiness to learn increase, the amount of external structuring decreases.

(d) *Sensory-motor deficits.* A not uncommon observation of the hyperactive child concerns the child's clumsiness. The child may experience a variety of sensory-motor problems, such as visual-perceptual or visual-motor difficulties. The psychoeducational treatment of hyperactivity usually includes an examination of the child's sensory-motor functioning. Subsequent programing will consider the child's sensory-motor profile, in terms of remediating the deficits or developing teaching procedures that circumvent the child's difficulties.

The two case studies in this chapter are illustrative of these considerations. They both involve extensive diagnostic efforts, followed by intervention programs aimed at remediating deficits, facilitating school learning, and managing the symptoms of hyperactivity.

References

CRUICKSHANK, W. M., BENTZEN, F. A., RATZBURG, F., and TANNHAUSER, M. T. *A Teaching Method for Brain-Injured and Hyperactive Children*. Syracuse: Syracuse University Press, 1961.

DOUGLAS, V. Stop, look and listen: The problem of sustained attention and impulse control in hyperactive and normal children. *Canadian J. Behav. Sci.* 1972, 4: 259-282.

DYCK, N. J. Educational management of hyperactive children. In Fine, M. J. (ed.), *Principle and Techniques of Intervention with Hyperactive Children*. Springfield, Ill.: Charles C Thomas, 1977.

FREIBERGS, V. and DOUGLAS, V. Concept learning in hyperactive and normal children. *J. Abnorm. Psychol.* 1969, 74:388-395.

HEWETT, F. Educational programs for children with behavior disorders. In Quay, H., and Werry, J. (eds.), *Psychopathological Disorders of Childhood*. New York: Wiley, 1972.

KEOGH, B. Hyperactivity and learning disorders: review and speculation. *Except. Child.* 1971, 38:101-110.

CASE STUDY #11. PSYCHOEDUCATIONAL PROGRAMMING WITH A HYPERACTIVE CHILD

Eunice Nelson

Current Problem

In a report to the psychologist, the following observations were made by the teacher: Anthony, age eight years, two months, moves constantly and is not responsive to correction or guidance. He is pleasant and friendly to both peers and adults. However, he does not get along with his peers because of his constant motion and short attention span.

Background Information

This child had a history of high-level physical activity and his pediatrician had diagnosed him hyperactive. He had been in a perceptual/motor training program due to organic eye problems and had a hearing loss, which resulted in ear surgery at the age of three. However, the hearing loss was considered to be minimal. Anthony had stomach surgery at the age of two, prior to which his stomach had been pumped twice at the age of one.

Anthony's mother was 16-years of age and his father was 19 when he was born. The mother had a history of severe allergies. Both parents, while seeming to be very immature, were quite concerned about their son's problems. They themselves seemed very hyperactive, which led the psychologist to consider how much of Anthony's behavior was modeling.

Anthony's father was a backyard mechanic and, during vacation, Anthony spent days at a time with his father, dismantling and assembling motors. His parents said he was able to concentrate on these tasks for long periods of time.

At age six, Anthony had been referred to a private counseling service for testing. During this testing, Anthony was distractible and inattentive, running about the room and climbing on the furniture. He made some attempt at performance of the testing tasks, but could not remain attentive. The psychologist was unable to complete any of the testing. His scores on the WISC-R were Verbal IQ, 79; Performance IQ, 60; and Full Scale IQ, 68. However, these scores were not considered valid.

The school psychologist observed Anthony in the classroom over a period of two weeks. He found Anthony to be immature, frustrated, and aggressive. Anthony had not separated his behaviors from himself; he considered himself to be an innately "bad boy," and had been so labeled by his peers. His distorted self-concept allowed him to take an inferior position when challenged, since he assumed he would fail in most situations.

While some of Anthony's hyperactivity may have been organic in origin, the psychologist felt that much of it was avoidance behavior. He noted that Anthony looked at the contract designed for him on occasion, but refused to attempt any of the tasks. On many days, he totally ignored his contract, even though the teacher had designed simple tasks for him. However, paper and pencil tasks required too much concentration, and the auditory programs were too confining. So, Anthony bounced about the room, like a rubber ball, leaving a path of chaos.

The psychologist suggested some changes be made in both the classroom environment and Anthony's treatment program. The teacher, in consultation with the psychologist, implemented the following intervention.

Intervention

Environmental modification followed the plan of Hewett's engineered classroom, with some slight variations (Hewett, 1974). The mastery and achievement center included the student's desks where Anthony, along with other students, carried out their contract assignments. Next to the desks were the more isolated "offices" for use by the students in order to reduce self-stimulation and fantasy preoccupation. As suggested by Hewett, the exploratory center was set behind the mastery center, in order to be less distracting. The exploratory center included science activities, filmstrips, slides, and games for reinforcement of academic skills. This center was also secluded, in order to be less distracting for Anthony, as well as for the other students. In order to maintain some control of Anthony's hyperactivity and distractability, he was given his own office, which was to become known as his "shop."

The next step in Anthony's treatment involved his academic program. Up to this point in his education, Anthony's program had been a hit-and-miss operation—mostly, miss. At the suggestion of the psychologist, all academic tasks were removed from Anthony's program, and the teacher asked Anthony to help her plan his contract on a day-to-day basis. She agreed to make concessions, if he would agree to some classroom rules. Anthony understood that any time he broke their agreement, his contract would be removed and he would be placed in the "time-out" booth. Being isolated from the group was a very aversive reinforcer for Anthony. However, it had been used infrequently and inconsistently in the past.

Anthony knew what he wished to have included in his contract. The teacher had not been especially innovative in using Anthony's mechanical abilities in his treatment. Anthony asked that he be allowed to set up the learning machines in the morning and take them down at night as a part of his contract. He also asked to load the slide and film projectors. None of the children had been allowed to do this, because of prior damage done to films, filmstrips, and slides. Anthony proved himslef to be an efficient and responsible operator. He dragged out a box of broken and battered miniature toys, which in the past had been used as reinforcers, and asked to repair them— also, a part of his contract. This was when his office became his shop and was the turning point in Anthony's educational program. The teacher's ingenuity was taxed to improvise tasks, related to Anthony's contract activities, that would help him learn the skills basic to reading, writing, spelling, and math. However, an old typewriter, which was placed in Anthony's shop, eventually became an invaluable tool. Anthony ignored the typewriter until he discovered the numbers. He was then seen to spend much time pecking away at the numbers. It was only after much success at math activities using the typewriter that Anthony could be persuaded to explore the letters (Figures 1 and 2).

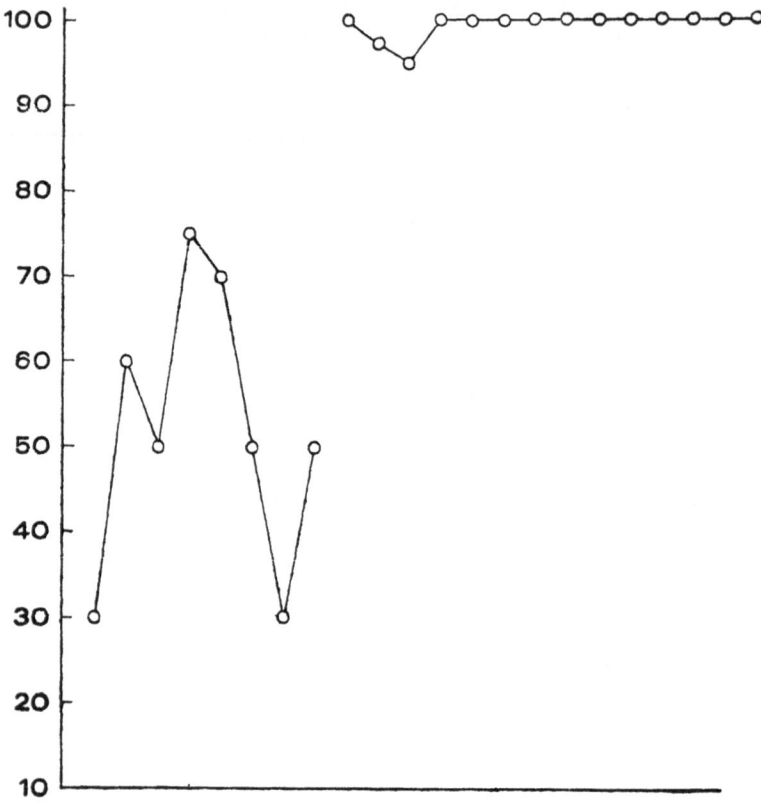

FIGURE 1. Percentage of addition problems completed correctly.
Reinforcement: points toward free time in his shop.

It was the consensus of both the psychologist and the teacher that class-room management of Anthony's behavior, both academic and social, was needed before he could be taught necessary academic skills. Early attempts at charting were futile. Only after much trial and error and many starts and stops was the valid charting illustrated in this text implemented.

A token economy was already in operation in the classroom. It had not been effective for Anthony, however, since he displayed few behaviors that could be rewarded.

As Anthony began to complete his contract assignments and receive tokens for his work, as did the other children, he began to ask for more work. His hyperactivity was diminishing (Figures 3 and 4). But, best of all, he was becoming a favorite with the other children in the room. As a rein-

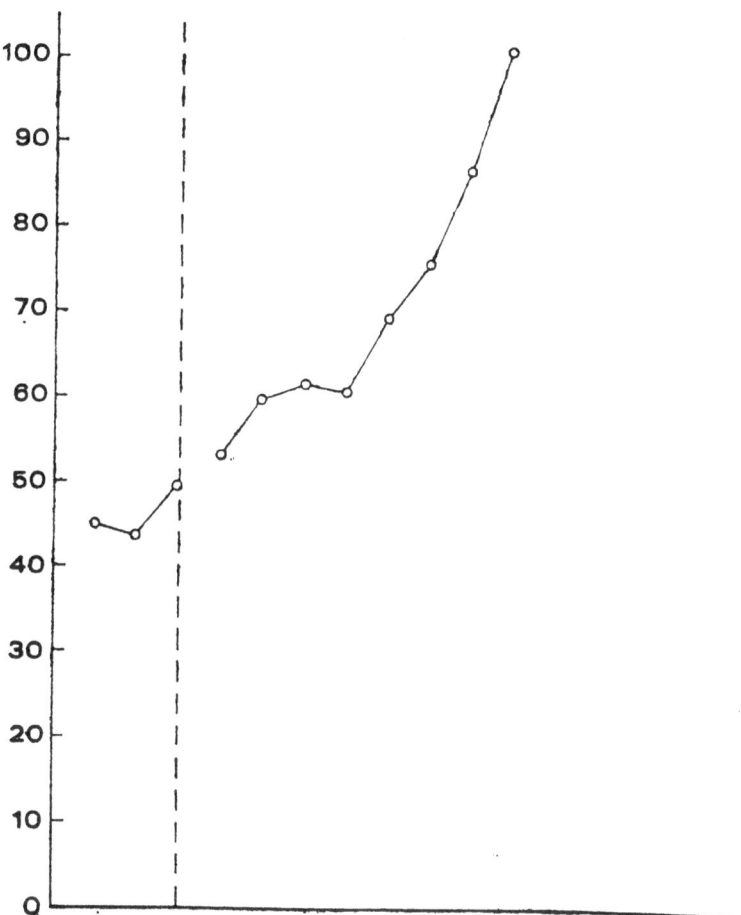

FIGURE 2. Completed addition facts on three-minute test.
Reinforcer: points toward free time in his shop.

forcer for completed contracts, a child could choose to be Anthony's helper. This was often negotiated between Anthony and prospective helpers, with the teacher acting as mediator.

It was now time to come to grips with Anthony's reading problem. Since he had been placed in a low-level math program, he was told that he could use the typewriter if he worked only with the letters. He refused to use the typewriter for several weeks, although he was seen to stand for minutes at a time gazing at the keyboard. One morning, upon arriving early to set up the machines, the teacher asked him how he would like to have a helper in his

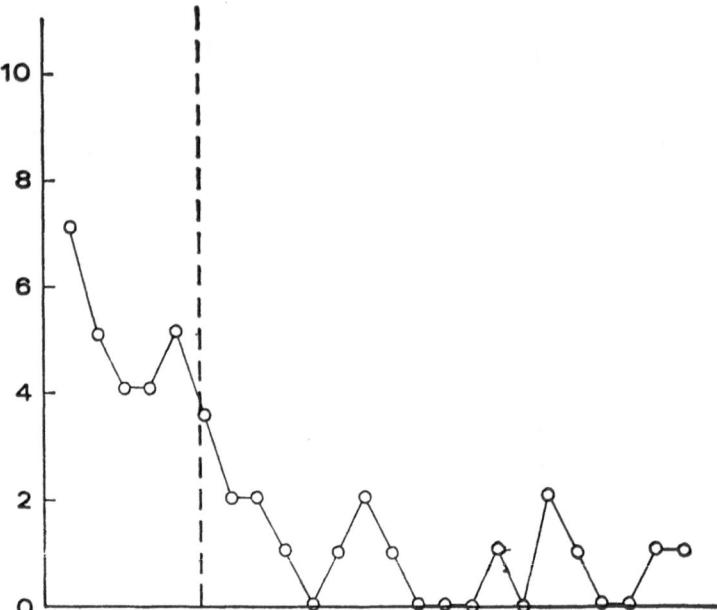

FIGURE 3. Incidence of talking without raising hand.
Reinforcement: points toward free time in his shop.

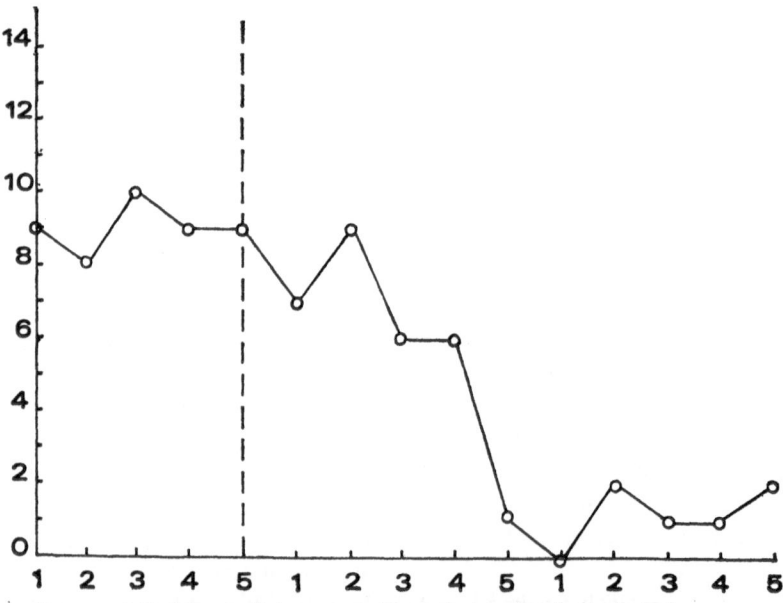

FIGURE 4. Incidence of times out-of-seat during 30-minute period.
Reinforcement: points toward free time in his shop.

shop to work "for" him at the typewriter. This solved some of Anthony's problem; he would now receive consistent support.

Recognizing and remembering the letters of the alphabet was difficult for Anthony, but not nearly so difficult as learning to read (Figure 5). He became interested in making words and copied words that he saw around the room. Each time Anthony copied a word, he asked the teacher or the aide to pronounce it. The teacher took this opportunity to build a sight vocabulary. However, Anthony became discouraged with his slow progress and began to regress. He could spell, but he could not read. Most authorities agree that, until a child learns to read, it is unlikely he will learn to spell. Anthony was an exception.

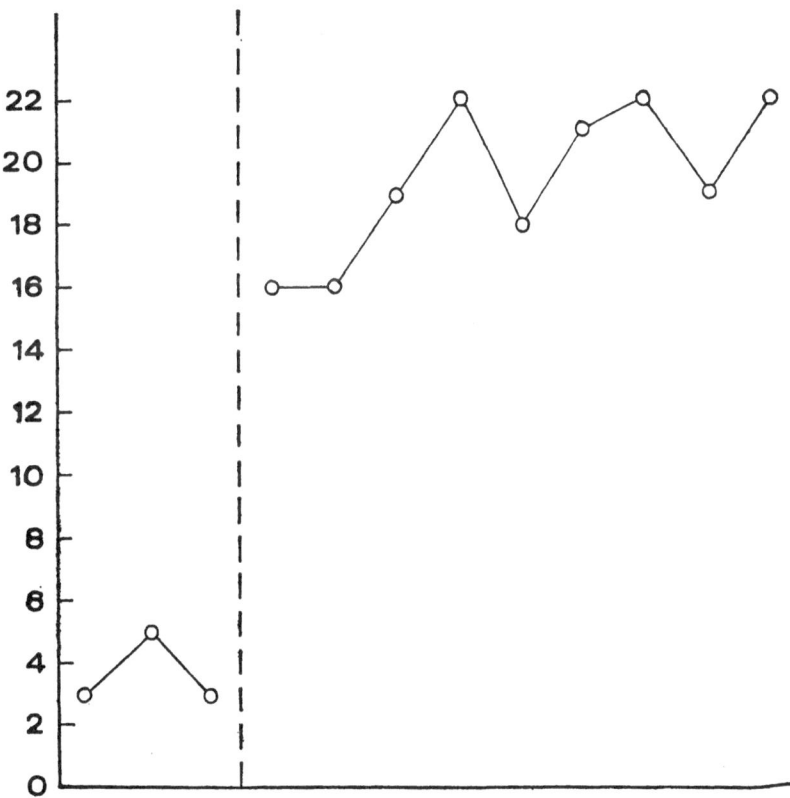

FIGURE 5. Incidence of correctly identified letters.
Reinforcement: points toward free time in his shop.

The teacher knew that until Anthony had a complete psychoeducational diagnosis, further attempts to teach him to read would be fruitless. Anthony had shown himself capable of concerted effort for relatively longer periods of time. The psychologist was again consulted and a plan for beginning the testing was implemented. It was determined that the teacher would administer the academic tests, and the psychologist would administer the other tests he deemed appropriate. Anthony was successful and moving into increasingly more difficult math concepts. In order to insure a successful experience in his first test experience, a math test was given. He was excited with the prospect of being able to show how well he could do on the test. He was very confident of his performance in math and often helped the other children in the room. He was elated when his test score showed him to be 2.6 years above his grade level (Table 1).

The teacher made observations using the Pupil Rating/Scale (Myklebust, 1971). "Fall-out" was noted in the auditory channel. This spurred the psychologist's testing of auditory processing and psycholinguistic development, in addition to tests of intellectual functioning and aptitude.

It became apparent that much depended on the expertise of the tester, in order to successfully complete the psychoeducational diagnosis. If Anthony became aware of any failure, it was feared that he would immediately revert to his hyperactive behavior in order to avoid the test situation. He often still used this avoidance behavior in the classroom.

The teacher and the psychologist were in agreement as to Anthony's capabilities in visual/motor areas. However, the Developmental Test of Visual Motor Integration (Beery and Butenica, 1967) as shown in Table 1, was administered by the psychologist, in order to lend credibility to teacher observation. Anthony had a VMI age of 11 years, which was approximately three years above his chronological age. Again, he was successful in the test situation and was becoming more and more interested in the testing. He became a willing subject and often asked how he was doing, wanting to know if his responses were right or wrong. The psychologist explained that all the answers were right for purposes of finding out everything he could about Anthony. Like in putting a puzzle together, the psychologist explained, there are no wrong pieces; all of them are right. They just have to be put in the right places to complete the puzzle. This seemed to satisfy Anthony, and he accepted the idea that he was like a puzzle with many right pieces.

The psychologist then administered the ITPA (Kirk et al., 1968), which showed weakness in auditory processing (Table 1).

The greatest testing hurdle was yet to be made, since it was time to administer the reading test. Here again, much depended on the expertise of the tester. The Basic Educational Skills Inventory was used (Adamson et al., 1972). Level A was administered in order to again give Anthony a successful test experience, as well as to provide a profile of strengths upon which to build a reading program (Table 1). Anthony was above criterion on all subtests with the exception of the sight word test. The teacher then proceeded with level B of the BESI (Figure 6). She used this as a criterion reference test, in order to maintain specificity in treatment. Those subtests were selected which were most appropriate as they related to the scope and sequence of skills. From fall-out in those subtests, prescriptive teaching was implemented in reading.

Following the psychoeducational testing, a second phase of intervention occurred. At this point, the treatment of Anthony's reading problem placed emphasis entirely on visual processing of reading tasks. Since Anthony's processing dysfunction was in the auditory channel, he could not learn to read by the phonics method, which had been used. Anthony was given visual cues to help him read and a linguistic approach to reading was implemented. Also, since he was progressing in math, most of the intervention time was devoted to reading and spelling.

Conclusion

Due to the personally and socially disruptive effects of Anthony's hyperactivity, he had fallen progressively farther behind in his school work. The psychologist had noted that his hyperactivity decreased when he was engaged in "backyard mechanics" with his father. It was suggested by the psychologist that this, in some way, be used as a catalyst to bring Anthony's hyperactivity under control. The "shop" (Anthony's suggestion) was used for this purpose. As his attention span increased (due to his interest in the shop activities), he became more and more productive in academic tasks related to "shop" activities. This was gradually extended to include other academic tasks outside the shop. Increase in productivity may be noted in Figures 1, 2, and 5. Deceleration of hyperactive behavior may be noted in Figures 3 and 4. The increased attention span and the decreased distractibility enabled Anthony to make the gains on the WRAT shown in Table 1.

Anthony is now able to work in the regular classroom for part of the day. When he cannot tolerate the regular classroom, he is allowed to return to the Learning Disabilities classroom to work on his assignments. He often

TABLE 1

Test Data

Subject: Anthony. Entered present school at age 7 years and 9 months. Referred to the psychologist at age 8 years and 2 months.

Testing done by the psychologist as follows:

ITPA	SS	C.A. 8-2 M.A. 7-9 P.L.A. 7-7
Auditory Reception	42	
Visual Memory	40	
Auditory Association	26	
Auditory Memory	26	
Visual Association	34	
Verbal Expression	24	
Grammatic Closure	18	
Manual Expression	40	
Auditory Closure	21	
Sound Blending	25	

Developmental Test of Visual Motor Integration
VMI Raw Score   19
VMI Age Equivalent   10 years 11 months

Testing done by the teacher as follows:
BASIC EDUCATIONAL SKILLS INVENTORY—LEVEL A

Memory for Sentences	3/22	
Direction in Space	10/10	
Same or Different	10/10	
Naming the Alphabet	26/26	
Printing Capital Letters of the Alphabet	52/52	
Printing Small Letters of the Alphabet	19/26	
Naming Manuscript Printed Letters	26/26	
Match Manuscript Letters of the Alphabet	11/11	
Naming Cursive Letters	23/26	
Sight Words	0/112	Stopped test after 10 consecutive errors.

BASIC EDUCATIONAL SKILLS INVENTORY—LEVEL B

Rhyming	4/10
Initial Consonant and Vowel Sounds	3/23
Final Consonant Sounds	0/10
Auditory Blending of Words	0/8
Initial Consonant Sounds	0/22

Wide Range Achievement Test-Pretest
Anthony—Age 8-6

TABLE 1 (continued)

The pretest on the WRAT was not considered valid due to the inability of Anthony to attend to the task. The grade equivalent scores on this test ranged from 1.6 to spelling to N.8 in reading and 1.9 in math.

Wide Range Achievement Test-Post-Test After Intervention: 2nd Phase
Anthony—Age 9-2

Reading Score	43	Grade Score	2.3	S.S.	83	Percentile	13
Spelling Score	28	Grade Score	2.2	S.S.	98	Percentile	7
Arithmetic Score	37	Grade Score	5.5	S.S.	107	Percentile	68

takes the initiative, when this is necessary. From the progress that Anthony has made, his prognosis for a successful school experience seems more likely.

References

ADAMSON, G., SHRAGO, M., and VAN ETTEN, G. *Basic Educational Skills Inventory.* Torrence, Calif.: Brad Winch Associates, 1972.

BEERY, K. E. and BUKTENICA, N. A. *Developmental Test of Visual-Motor Integration.* Chicago: Follett Educational Corporation, 1967.

HEWETT, F. M. and FORENESS, S. R. *Education of Exceptional Learners.* Boston: Allyn & Bacon, Inc., 1974.

KIRK, S. A., MCCARTHY, J. J., and KIRK, W. *Illinois Test of Psycholinguistic Abilities.* Urbana, Ill.: University of Illinois Press, 1968.

MYKLEBUST, H. R. *The Pupil Rating Scale.* New York: Grune & Stratton, Inc., 1971.

CASE STUDY #12. USE OF A STRUCTURED CLASSROOM APPROACH WITH A MULTISENSORY INSTRUCTIONAL STRATEGY

Fred H. Wallbrown

Current Problem

Referral and Classroom Observation

At the request of the principal of his school, Ron was first seen by the school psychologist on an emergency basis during the first week of November. The first step in the assessment procedure consisted of the pyschologist's observing Ron's behavior in the classroom. The observation lasted for approximately one hour, until the principal was free to take over the class so that the teacher could consult with the psychologist. During the observation period, a pattern of overactivity, distractibility, impulsiviy, motoric awkwardness, and general classroom disruption was evident in Ron's behavior. He left his seat 17 times during this period and did not return until the teacher stopped what she was doing and ordered him back to his seat.

A pattern soon emerged while the psychologist was observing Ron's behavior. It became evident that when Ron left his seat, he did so when his attention was attracted by some form of extraneous auditory stimuli, such as the sounds made from crunching a sheet of paper, dropping a pencil, sharpening a pencil, activity in a reading group, noises in the hall, or the sounds of other children moving around the room. His usual pattern was to leave his seat and start moving toward the source of the noise. However, the noise which originally attracted Ron did not keep his attention for long, and he became distracted by some other sound. For example, on one occasion Ron first left his seat and started moving toward another child who had crunched a sheet of paper. As Ron was walking toward this child's desk, the voice inflection of the teacher changed as she uttered an enthusiastic exclamation while working with her reading group. When the teacher's voice quality changed, Ron immediately stopped, focused his attention on the teacher, and then started toward the reading group. On the way toward the group, Ron tripped over another child's foot and fell in the aisle, making a loud noise and knocking objects off of adjacent desks.

At this point, the teacher stood up and, in a strong voice, ordered Ron back to his seat by exclaiming, "Ron! Go back to your seat and stay there!" Ron seemed confused and did not respond immediately. The teacher walked over to him, took him by the arm, walked him briskly back to his seat, and placed him in it. Before departing, she gave Ron a firm glance and in a stern voice said, "Stay in your seat and don't disturb the other boys and girls!" Ron put his head down on the desk and remained quiet for three or four minutes, but he was soon kicking the desk of the child in front of him.

Another aspect of Ron's behavior pattern became evident in the course of the observation. Even though Ron was especially distractible by extraneous noises, it became clear that movement was the one kind of visual stimuli that could sustain his attention. This tendency first became evident when the psychologist noted that Ron's attention was focused intently on the teacher as she was talking to the class and at the same time writing on the chalkboard, gesturing in an animated fashion, and moving around in front of the class. This aspect of Ron's behavior pattern was confirmed by other incidents when Ron sustained his attention on movements of the teacher or other children in the class. Ron did not leave his seat when someone was moving around in the class. In addition, there was a clear-cut decrease in extraneous motoric activities such as seat kicking, pencil tapping, dropping objects, and hitting other children while Ron was following movement in his visual field. Further observation indicated that Ron was less likely to be distracted by extraneous classroom noises while he was following movement in his visual field.

Teacher Consultation

The second step in assessing the situation and defining the problem consisted of consultation with the teacher concerning Ron's learning pattern and classroom behavior. The behavior pattern described by the teacher was in general agreement with the behaviors observed by the school psychologist, allowing for the emotionality and anger occasioned by the frustration she had encountered in working with Ron. It soon became evident that the teacher perceived Ron's chronic pattern of disruptive behavior as a threat to her control of the class. The following are examples of the disruptive behaviors described by the teacher: "won't stay in his seat . . . wanders around the room bothering other children . . . won't do his work . . . hits other children . . . marks up other children's papers and tries to tear up their things . . . runs into other children and falls over everything . . . doesn't pay attention . . . won't finish anything . . . won't follow directions . . . just doesn't try . . . isn't making any progress." The teacher's comments indicated that she was thoroughly exasperated with Ron and felt that he should be placed in a special class or be put back into kindergarten.

Further conversation with the teacher indicated that she had invested a great deal of effort in working with Ron and communicating with his parents. Some of the strategies she tried included ignoring disruptive behavior and reinforcing positive behavior with verbal praise, food, toys, tokens, and special privileges. At other times, the teacher indicated, she had used punishment such as sending Ron to the principal's office, scolding him verbally, and moving him out into the hall to work. Other efforts included trying to reason with him at various times, as well as keeping him in during recess and after school, as punishment for not finishing his work or some form of misbehavior in the classroom. The teacher also mentioned that when she sent worksheets home with Ron, at the request of his parents, he usually brought them back to school completed, but could not do the same kind of work in school the next day.

Background Information

Information Gained from School Personnel

The teacher reported that Ron came a middle-class family that had an active interest in his school progress. His father was employed as an engineer, and his mother was a housewife who devoted most of her time to caring for a three-year-old son, but was actively involved in church work and civic activities. An older son from the family was making excellent progress in third grade and was reportedly popular and well liked by his teachers and peers. All of the teacher's contacts with the family indicated that the parents were compatible, happily married, and in good financial condition.

The teacher did note, however, that Ron's parents had been adamantly opposed to having him retained in kindergarten when his previous teacher had suggested the idea and pointed out his general immaturity, poor readiness skills, short attention span, distractibility, and inability to sit still and remain in his seat. In recent conversations with the teacher, the parents had expressed the same feelings and based their argument on the fact that Ron was already older than most children in the class (CA = 7-0), as well as larger than most of his classmates. The father consistently expressed the opinion that strict discipline would teach Ron that he had to behave himself and work in school rather than play around. At the same time, the father indicated that the teacher should feel free to spank Ron or keep him after school if he misbehaved or failed to complete his school work.

The parents had informed a school counselor that they had already discussed Ron's difficulties with their pediatrician. The pediatrician informed them that he could not find anything physically wrong with Ron but he did observe that he was a "little overactive and has a short attention span." The pediatrician had also advised the parents to "have the school psychologist check Ron to see if he has a learning disability."

Psychological Assessment

The parents readily agreed to a psychological assessment when they were contacted by the school counselor for their permission and signature on the consent form. A battery of standardized, individual tests were administered over three different sessions, scheduled on different days. On the Wechsler Intelligence Scale for Children—Revised, Ron earned the following configuration of scaled scores on the twelve subtests: Information, 13; Similarities, 14; Arithmetic, 6; Vocabulary, 13; Comprehension, 14; Digit Span, 6;

Picture Completion, 7; Picture Arrangement, 10; Block Design, 12; Object Assembly, 12; Coding, 7; and Mazes, 12. The Full Scale IQ from the WISC-R was 108, whereas the Verbal IQ was 112 and the Performance IQ was 96. On the Peabody Picture Vocabulary Test (form A), Ron received an IQ of 122 and an MA of 9-2. In addition, Ron received a standard score (comparable to IQ) of 87 on the Draw-A-Person (scored with Good-enough-Harris standards), but he took only 52 seconds to complete his drawing of a man.

Several tentative conclusions were suggested from Ron's performance on the three ability tests mentioned above. First, it was evident that Ron possessed the scholastic aptitude/general intelligence necessary for mastery of the basic skills included in the first-grade curriculum. Second, the configuration of the IQ scores from the ability tests (PPVT > WISC-R > DAP) is typical of what is ordinarily obtained for hyperactive children with an attentional deficit. Third, a low score on the Freedom From Distractibility factor (Arithmetic and Digit Span from the WISC-R) not only indicated that Ron had difficulty screening out extraneous noises and concentrating on the essential elements of a task, but also suggested a poor auditory memory (short-term) for non-meaningful material (that which cannot be meaningfully organized in some fashion). Fourth, the short working time for the DAP, as well as observation while Ron was making his drawing, suggested that he had an impulsive cognitive style. Fifth, interaction with Ron during the evaluation indicated that he was a verbal child capable of expressing his thoughts with precision, fluency, and clarity.

Standardized measures of perceptual development, linguistic development, and achievement skills were also included in the assessment. In this regard, Ron completed his reproduction of the Bender designs in 2' 11" and his total Koppitz score was 14. No outstanding pattern was evident in Ron's errors on the Bender. Rather, observation of how the designs were produced and the qualitative aspects of the error pattern indicated an impulsive cognitive style, as well as a gross deficit in visual-motor integration. Scores from the Wepman Auditory Discrimination Test (form II) suggested an attentional deficit for auditory stimuli, but failed to provide conclusive information concerning auditory discrimination skills. On this test, the X-score was 12 and the Y-score was 4, when the test was administered in accordance with the standard directions. When Ron was allowed to turn around and face the examiner during limits testing, the number of X-errors was reduced to 3 and the Y-errors to 0 on form I of the Wepman.

Several subtests from the Illinois Test of Psycholinguistic Abilities were also included in the assessment battery, but they failed to provide much additional information about Ron's learning pattern. Standard scores for the ITPA subtests were as follows: Auditory Reception, 34; Auditory Closure, 30; Auditory Association, 42; Visual Sequential Memory, 33; and Visual Closure, 31.

Analysis of Ron's responses to the Wide Range Achievement Test and informal assessment procedures indicated an uneven, erratic pattern of achievement skills. On the Arithmetic subtest, Ron earned a grade-equivalent score of Kdg. 0.6 (SS = 76). In terms of skills, this score reflects the fact that Ron was able to count meaningfully from 1 to 15, recognize the numerals 3 and 5, hold up 3 and 8 fingers on command, and recognize that 9 is greater than 6. In contrast, Ron was not able to complete any of the written problems successfully or respond correctly to any of the three mental arithmetic problems. Informal assessment indicated that Ron could count objects meaningfully from 1 through 25 or 26, but could not associate quantities with numerals beyond 4 or 5. Similarly, Ron could write most of the numerals from 1 to 10, but, beyond 5 or 6, he often confused their names and sequence. Reversals were also common in Ron's reproductions of the numerals 2, 3, 4, 7, and 9.

On the Word Recognition subtest of the WRAT, Ron received a grade-equivalent score of Kdg. 0.1 (SS = 69). He earned this score on the basis of being able to match 5 out of 10 letters (A, R, Z, S, E) with the same letters in another row, name 3 of 13 letters (A, B, R), and name the first letter in his own name. On this subtest, Ron was not able to recognize any of the words or name any of the letters of his own name beyond the first one. However, Ron was able to recite his "ABC's" verbally and made only four errors in doing so (omissions of O, P, T, U).

Informal assessment procedures indicated that Ron's oral comprehension was good and that his auditory memory for meaningful material was adequate. When Ron's attention was maintained through physical contact (examiner's hand on Ron's back or shoulder with firm grasp; examiner's knee against Ron's thigh), he was able to answer questions on short passages read to him and repeat relatively complex sentences presented orally to him. Requiring Ron to maintain eye contact with the examiner facilitated his performance during this part of the assessment.

Intervention

The school psychologist, teacher, counselor, and reading teacher met together and developed an intervention program for Ron. This staff conference occurred after the school psychologist and teacher had met with the parents and discussed Ron's learning and behavior pattern with them. The parents were able to understand the information presented to them and not only requested reading material about the area of learning disabilities, but also offered to help by working with Ron at home. At the time of the conference, however, the parents expressed disapproval of any type of placement in a learning-disabilities class, so it was necessary to develop the intervention around Ron's participation in regular classroom activities.

The intervention program developed for Ron in the case conference included two major areas of focus. The first area of concern was helping the teacher develop an effective classroom management program based on available information about Ron's learning and behavior patterns. The second area of concern involved preparing an instructional strategy most appropriate for Ron's particular learning pattern. These two aspects of the intervention strategy are discussed separately in the present section, since the management program was implemented primarily within the confines of the classroom. The primary thrust of the instructional strategy, however, was implemented through individual tutoring on a one-to-one basis outside the confines of the regular classroom.

Classroom Management

Since Ron's hyperactivity and distractibility were the salient constraints to effective classroom learning, the focus of the case conference was on determining management procedures to bring these behaviors under control. The fundamental issue seemed to involve controlling the amount of environmental stimulation, in both the auditory and visual learning modes. It was agreed upon by the group that the custodian should be asked to construct a small study carrel for Ron to use while he was working individually on seat-work activities. The purpose of the study carrel was to control extraneous visual stimuli (especially movement). One of the group members suggested that a set of earphones should be obtained to protect Ron from the influence of extraneous classroom noises.

The final arrangement consisted of three small 30″ × 36″ study carrels constructed of Masonite, with a 2″ × 4″ frame that was fastened solidly to the floor. The sides of the carrels were sufficiently high so that a student could not see over the top while standing. The size of the carrels was limited, since there was some reason to believe that a smaller space inhibits hyperactivity. A pastel color, similar to the color of the classroom walls, was used to paint the carrels.

It was the teacher's idea to construct three carrels, rather than only one for Ron. Several considerations probably influenced the teacher's request for additional carrels, but her most persuasive argument was that she had other students who, from time to time, could benefit from having a private place to study, away from the rest of the class. With this arrangement, the teacher reasoned that working in a private carrel could be made into a special privilege rather than something that singled Ron out from the rest of the class. While the carrels were being constructed, the teacher followed through with her idea by explaining to the class that the carrels were "a special place for boys and girls to work when bothered by the noise in our class." The teacher's argument for additional carrels was fully justified. Working in the carrels became popular with the entire class immediately and several children showed a continued preference for working in the carrels throughout the entire school year.

In Ron's case, the study carrel was used only during those times when he was required to engage in independent activities, such as worksheets, exercises, or other forms of seat-work. Consequently, it was still necessary for those persons participating in the staffing to help the teacher develop a strategy for structuring Ron's behavior during large and small group instruction. Here, the assessment data indicated that physical contact had a settling effect on Ron's activity level and attentional process. As a result, participants in the case conference focused on how this information could be used in a group setting.

The following suggestions were generated and incorporated into the management strategy: (1) For large group instruction, Ron's seat should be moved up beside the teacher's desk, so that he would be close enough to her to have frequent physical contact during large group instruction; (2) For reading group (initially readiness group), Ron was to be moved so that was beside the teacher and she could maintain extensive physical contact (arm around him, and firm grip on shoulder or arm); and (3) During large and small group instruction, the teacher should insist that Ron maintain eye contact with her while she was speaking.

Since the assessment data indicated that Ron tended to orient himself immediately to novel sounds, the staffing group concentrated on determining how the teacher could use this information to manage his classroom behavior more effectively. Several possibilities were generated. First, the group suggested that Ron could become the teacher's helper and she could allow him to repeat back the directions which she had just given to the class. The teacher felt that this suggestion was helpful. She decided that it would be a good idea with the entire class, making sure that Ron was allowed to be the helper frequently. The group further noted that this suggestion should also be helpful in checking Ron's impulsive tendency to rush into work before getting the directions straight. Second, the group suggested that the teacher should simply call out Ron's name with emphasis (cueing) when she observed that he was not paying attention during large or small group interaction. Third, the group suggested that the teacher should practice using different inflections, variations in voice quality, and pauses, and observe how these influenced Ron's attention. This suggestion made sense to the teacher and she also indicated that she would monitor the pacing of her verbal directions and explanations to the class.

Another finding from the assessment was that movement tended to hold Ron's attention extremely well and help him tune out extraneous noises. On the basis of this information, the group suggested that the teacher make a deliberate attempt to emphasize movement during large group instruction. The group also suggested that the teacher concentrate on expanding her range of hand gestures, head movements, and body posturing while working with small groups as well as the entire class. In the course of this discussion, the group generated many specific examples that the teacher might use; e.g., hand motions to express large, small, short, tall, near, distant, around, over, below, beside, out, and in. Other suggestions included such activities as tracing letters and numbers in the air while discussing them verbally, and a wide array of gestures for action words.

Finally, the teacher noted that Ron seemed to become upset, agitated, and overactive when he was presented with something new, unusual, or surprising. From this information, the group proceeded to discuss ways that the teacher could go about helping Ron establish and maintain regularity in his classroom environment. It was decided that for a while the teacher should have Ron come into the classroom a few minutes early and go over the activities for the day with him. This procedure was to continue until Ron memorized the sequence of activities which ordinarily occurred in the course of a regular day's activities. After the routine was mastered, it was decided that Ron should check with the teacher after school to determine if anything unusual was to happen the next day.

Instructional Strategy

The results of the assessment provided a substantial amount of information which was used in planning an instructional strategy for Ron. The first consideration by persons attending the staffing was that the teaching method selected should be the one most appropriate for a hyperactive child who is highly distractible by extraneous noises and movement. The staffing group was also very concerned that the method selected be appropriate for Ron's deficit in short-term auditory memory for non-meaningful material. The impulsivity noted earlier, as well as the difficulties with visual-motor integration, fine motor coordination, and gross motor coordination were also considered by the group. During the staffing, the teacher added information from her recent observations that indicated directional confusion was another area of difficulty for Ron.

Based on these considerations, the staffing group decided that a multi-sensory instructional strategy, with an emphasis on repetition, would be the most appropriate for Ron. Several methods were considered but, for several reasons, the group ultimately decided on the Shedd system (Shedd, 1968; Shedd and Blankenship, 1967a; Shedd and Blankenship, 1967b). The primary reason that the Shedd approach was chosen over the alternative VAKT (visual-auditory-kinesthetic-tactual) system was because of its emphasis on repetition and drill that involves coordination of the kinesthetic and tactual learning modes. Second, the Shedd approach is highly structured, so that the student soon develops a routine which he is to follow throughout the program, regardless of how far he/she progresses. Third, the Shedd method utilizes cursive writing (rather than manuscript), which is most appropriate for use with hyperactive, distractible children. Fourth, the program developed by Shedd includes sequenced materials which were originally developed for multisensory instruction. The availability of these materials saved both the classroom teacher and remedial reading teacher from spending an inordinate amount of time in the planning and preparation of materials. Finally, the directions for use of the Shedd program are simple, straightforward and comprehensive, so it was possible for the reading teacher to show the parents how to use the method with Ron.

The reading teacher agreed to serve as the resource person and coordinate the overall instructional program for Ron, as well as provide 30 minutes of individual tutoring for him each day. The coordination included familiarizing the classroom teacher with the method and materials for the reading program, as well as showing her how to provide math instruction in accordance with the Shedd method. The teacher, in turn, agreed to allow Ron to use cursive writing in the classroom and make sure he followed through on the reading procedures learned in individual tutoring. In addition, the teacher agreed to provide Ron with at least three sessions of individual math tutoring (30 minutes per session) after school and as much extra help as time permitted during the regular school day. Finally, the reading teacher took the responsibility for showing the parents how to use the Shedd materials (math and reading) to help Ron at home, and supervising their work with him. The group decided that the parents should spend only 30 minutes (15 on math and 15 on reading) helping Ron with his school work each evening.

Remediation was initiated through use of the *Introductory Student's Manual,* which is the first book in the reading program developed by Shedd. The contents of this book cover the short vowel sounds, consonants, a few common diagraphs (wh, th, sh, and ch), and one sight words ("The"). With the Shedd method, the student is immediately introduced to the letter "a," shown in the printed from (lower and upper case), along with the cursive form (lower and upper case) of the letter. The tutor starts out by having the student learn the name of the letter "a" and its sound ("uh" in isolation and short vowel sound when combined with a consonant as in "ad," "as," or "hat"). Next, the student is required to trace the letter "a" on a model with the first finger of the preferred hand while saying its name. This process is repeated three times. In tracing over the visual letter model (in the book) the student begins with the dot and follows the arrows which indicate the proper strokes. The student is then required to trace the cursive form of the letter "a" on the rough side of a 12″ × 12″ Masonite board three times, while saying its name. After this, the student is required to write the letter "a" three times on a sheet of paper while saying its name. Also, the short vowel sound of the letter "a" is added and the student is required to repeat the reproduction procedure (model-Masonite-paper), while saying the short vowel sound of the letter.

The description above of teaching the letter "a" is abbreviated substantially, since 14 distinct steps are described in the teacher's manual. For example, the student is also required to think of other words with the same sound, combine "a" with "t" (the next letter to be learned), to make the word "at," read (from left to right) "at, a, at, a, a, at . . ." and learn the name of the letter coming directly after "a" in the alphabet. If the student makes an error at any time during this process, he/she is shown the appropriate response and required to continue until the response is correctly repeated three times.

The consonants "t," "p," "h," "c," "n," are similarly introduced during the initial stage of the Shedd reading program. However, the student is taught to form and write the word "at" as soon as the first two letters, "a" and "t," are learned. The student also learns how two letters can be used to form a word family ("at") so that words like "pat," "hat," and "cat" can be formed as new consonants are learned. The process of forming new words and word families (phonograms) continues as the child moves along in this reading program. Spelling is an integral component of the program, and students gradually learn to take full sentence dictation as they move further along in the program.

Conclusion

In Ron's case, progress through the reading program was extremely rapid. Within two weeks, he was able to master the first six letters in the program ("a," "t," "p," "c," "n") so that he could read and write a large number of words such as "tap," "pan," "cat," "can," and short sentences such as "Tap at a can" and "Pat a cat." Ron's initial success with the Shedd reading program not only gave him a great deal of intrinsic satisfaction from his own sense of accomplishment, but also earned a great deal of extrinsic reinforcement from his parents, teacher, and reading teachers. Consequently, Ron was able to make rapid progress through the introductory book.

The major difficulty encountered in working with Ron consisted of keeping him from trying to go too fast and getting careless about keeping his arm lifted from the desk while writing, tracing accurately, and repeating incorrect responses for all three correct repetitions.

During the second week of March, the reading teacher decided to discontinue individual tutoring with Ron since he had successfully completed all of the introductory book and had been able to transfer his skills to the regular classroom setting. At this time, Ron had been transferred to the top reading group in his class and was functioning effectively there with regular instruction. Since progress in the area of arithmetic was much less dramatic, his parents were instructed to discontinue providing help in reading and concentrate on the arithmetic program.

The Wide Range Achievement Test was readministered to Ron near the end of May in order to evaluate his progress. On the Word Recognition subtest, his grade equivalent score was 2.7 (SS = 99) at this time. The teacher's opinion not only substantiated Ron's score for sight vocabulary, but also indicated a similar level of achievement for reading comprehension and word attack skills. The Spelling subtest was also administered at this time and Ron earned a grade-equivalent score of 2.5 (SS = 96). Ron's grade-equivalent score for the Arithmetic subtest was 1.6 (SS = 84), which substantiated the teacher's opinion that he was still considerably below average in this area.

The classroom management program developed for Ron also proved to be relatively successful. Use of the study carrel and earphones was successful in eliminating most of Ron's leaving his seat and wandering around the class disturbing others during the time when seatwork was assigned to his reading group.

Structuring Ron's behavior during large group instruction proved to be somewhat more difficult. However, the teacher reported that Ron's behavior was within tolerable bounds two weeks after the management program was initiated. Substantial progress in Ron's behavior was reported by the teacher throughout the remainder of the school year.

Three short follow-up conferences were routinely scheduled to check on Ron's progress in the program designed for him (after two weeks, six weeks, and near the end of the school year). The information reported above was obtained in these meetings, informal chats in the hall, a brief year-end evaluation, and consultation requested by the teacher during the five weeks immediately after the program was initiated. Probably the best evidence of the success of the program was that the teacher did not request further consultation after Ron had been in the new program for five weeks.

References

SHEDD, C. *Instructor's Manual for the APSL Approach to Literacy.* Birmingham, Ala.: Reading Disability Center and Clinic, University of Alabama Medical College, 1968.

SHEDD, C. and BLANKENSHIP, F. *Student's Manual for Introduction to the APSL Approach to Literacy.* Birmingham, Ala.: Reading Disability Center and Clinic, University of Alabama Medical College, 1967. (a)

SHEDD, C. and BLANKENSHIP, F. *Teacher's Manual for Introduction to the APSL Approach to Literacy.* Birmingham, Ala.: Reading Disability Center and Clinic, University of Alabama Medical College, 1967. (b)

CHAPTER 5

Perceptual-Motor Training

Perceptual-motor and motor problems have long been associated with the hyperactivity syndrome. In most texts describing the hyperactivity syndrome, mention is made of motor problems as at least a probable related symptom that can be troublesome for the child. Wender (1973) stated that approximately half of all hyperactive children reveal coordination difficulties.

Stewart and Olds (1973) and Wender (1973) described some of the day-to-day problems that motor awkwardness presents for the child. Especially for the younger child, buttoning, cutting with scissors, tying shoelaces, printing within the lines, and accurately reproducing letters can pose serious frustrations. The visual-perceptual side of perceptual-motor problems often is reflected in reversals such as "b" for "d." Peer acceptance and social relationships can be affected, as the child with motor or perceptual-motor problems is unable to compete favorably in sports.

The inception of the motor and perceptual-motor problems still remains speculative. For some, these problems are classified as "soft" signs, symptomatic of neurological difficulties. Terms such as "developmental lag" are often used to describe the apparent unevenness of development. The implication of this term seems to be that the child will eventually catch up or accelerate in that area of development. While development continues, and some of the problems such as letter reversals disappear, the awkward child does not often become the acclaimed athlete.

It should be noted that motor and visual-motor problems may not always exist simultaneously. Wender (1973) described the combinations of coordination problems that can occur. For example, in some instances, children with eye-hand coordination problems may perform adequately on tasks requiring large muscle groups. It seems to be the fine motor and perceptual motor areas that are most problematic for the hyperactive child (Weiss et al., 1971). Indeed, the greater the severity of hyperactivity, the greater seems to be the degree of visual-motor deficits (Loney et al., 1978). While perceptual-motor difficulties are problematic of themselves, they may also be indicative of more basic cognitive difficulties, with far-reaching effects on learning and social adjustment.

The case studies being presented in this chapter reflect extensive efforts at perceptual-motor training from a particular viewpoint. The rationale for the interventions are described and detailed lesson plans are also included.

References

LONEY, J., LANGHORNE, J. E., and PATERNITE, C. E. An empirical basis for subgrouping the hyperkinetic/minimal brain dysfunction syndrome. *J. Abnorm. Psychol.* 1978, 87:431-441.

STEWART, M. A. and OLDS, S. W. *Raising a Hyperactive Child.* New York: Harper & Row, 1973.

WEISS, G., MINDE, L., WERRY, J., DOUGLAS, V., and NEMETH, E. Hyperactive children—five years later. *Arch. Gen. Psychiat.* 1971, 24:409-414.

WENDER, P. H. *The Hyperactive Child: A Handbook for Parents.* New York: Crown Publishers, 1973.

CASE STUDY #13. PERCEPTUAL-MOTOR TRAINING WITH A FIVE-YEAR-OLD BOY

Jean Pypher

The majority of children admitted to the University of Kansas Perceptual-Motor Clinic demonstrate sensory-input system developmental lags. Sensory-input behaviors evaluated and worked with include tactile, kinesthetic, vestibular, reflex, and visual.

The most common type of tactile dysfunction seen is what is known as "tactile defensiveness." Tactile defensiveness is caused by a negative reaction to tactile stimuli that results in hyperactivity and extreme distractibility. Ayres and others (Ayres, 1974; de Quiros and Schrager, 1978) postulate that a lack of balance between the discriminative and protective cutaneous afferent systems creates a tactile set that causes pressure to the skin that is interpreted as unpleasant by the tactile defensive individual. Such people are reported to strongly resist being held and cuddled as infants (and as adults), have little tolerance for being toweled down after a bath, and are extremely active when dressed in turtleneck or long-sleeved sweaters.

Tactile defensiveness is identified through the use of single and double tactile stimulation techniques, such as those found in the Southern California Kinesthesia and Tactile Perception Tests (Ayres, 1972); however, the reader is cautioned that the reported validity and reliability of these tests, particularly with very young children, are quite low. Behavioral observations and parental reports of the child's reaction to tactile stimulation are very important in the diagnostic procedure.

Therapeutic intervention for the tactile defensive child includes pressure applied, along with cutaneous stimulation and training in conscious relaxation techniques. Initially, children are given opportunities to "brush" exposed areas of skin with textures varying from course to very fine. Clinical observations indicate the more hyperactive the tactile defensive child, the coarser the initial texture selected. As therapy progresses, selected textures vary and tolerance for lighter touch improves.

Length of intervention depends upon the reaction of the child. Some children's active behavior and distractibility are markedly reduced after two months of daily cutaneous stimulation; some children demonstrate a gradual calming over a two-year period.

A child is considered "normal" tactily when he passes the single- and double-point stimulation test (Southern California Battery), can attend to the task the same length of time as his normally developing peers, and can remain motionless during conscious relaxation for five continuous minutes.

The following case history represents one of the most challenging cases we have worked with. We selected this child to write about because, although neurologically sound, he functioned extremely low perceptually. In addition to being a classical tactile defensive hyperactive, he demonstrated several other sensory-input dysfunctions.

Our goal for the child, as for all youngsters we work with, is sensory-perceptual-motor behavior at a level consistent with normative standards for the child's age. We begin at the level the child is performing at and proceed along a normal developmental sequence. A variety of therapeutic techniques are used (Ayres, 1974; Bobath and Bobath, 1964; Frostig and Horne,

1964; Getman et al., 1968; Kephart, 1963; Stockmeyer, 1967) depending upon at what level of development the child is functioning. Progress is assessed every 3 to 4 months; modifications in programing are made at that time.

Current Problem

Bobby was the youngest member in a family of three boys. The next oldest boy, Bill, had been evaluated by the Perceptual-Motor Clinic, found to have rather extensive perceptual-motor problems, and admitted to the clinic for a therapeutic program. The parents, noticing that Bobby demonstrated many of the same characteristics as Bill, requested evaluation of their youngest child in the Fall of 1974. When tested, Bobby was just under five years of age. His parents estimated his problem to be one of auditory perception and fine motor.

Background Information

His parents reported that Bobby's pre-, peri-, and postnatal developmental histories were unremarkable. Prenatal care was begun in the third month of pregnancy, gestation was of normal length, and a labor of 1½ hours was not difficult. A local anesthesia was used with no birth complications. Bobby weighed 7 lbs., 9 oz. and was 20 inches long at birth. The parents' report noted that the youngster sat without support at 7 months, pulled himself up without assistance at 11 months, and walked at 14 months; however, he required assistance with buttoning, tying, zipping, lacing and buckling when referred for clinic evaluation. He did not speak in one and two-word sentences until age four.

Bobby was tested during two different evaluation sessions, each 1½ hours long and three days apart. The young boy was one of the most difficult children we have ever tested. He seemed unable to understand directions, whether they were given verbally or demonstrated, or he was passively manipulated into place. He showed no facial expression during testing and no response to verbal praise; if patted on the back or head, he pushed the examiner's hand away. An excessive amount of extraneous movement, such as head or hand shaking and kicking of legs when seated, was demonstrated throughout the testing periods. Test results indicated that Bobby demonstrated six primitive reflexes (these usually do not persist after the first year of life) and lacked five equilibrium reflexes. The tactile test results indicated that he was able to identify all single points of stimuli to the hand and cheek, however, when two-point stimulation first to the cheeks and then to the hands were applied, he perceived only the stimulus to the right side. When two-point stimuli were applied to the hand and cheek simultaneously, he perceived only those stimuli that touched the cheek. Both his visual and auditory attention spans were reported to be extremely brief; during visual tracking tasks he tended to move his head rather than his eyes. The child's static and dynamic balance performances, fine motor and hand-eye co-ordination were all well below expectations for his age group. He had diffi-culty with all directional movement on the balance beam, could not move between two objects without touching them, and would not touch body parts when asked to identify their location. His self drawing included a head, hair, eyes, trunk, mouth, and feet. He was unable to perform any of the finger-to-nose, finger-to-finger, or successive finger tasks. He had very little hand gripping strength.

Because of Bobby's unusually poor upper-limb strength and his inability to perform some of the finger-touch test items, we referred the child for neurological and psychological examinations. The neurologist reported that the physical examination was normal, except that the child winced when-ever the doctor moved. The doctor also reported that Bobby was not proficient in fine coordination, but he saw no abnormalities in coordination or evidence of any special neurological deficiency, except as it related to the child's delayed speech and general "clumsy" movements. The psychologist reported that the child was functioning overall within the borderline retardation range of intelligence (Wechsler norms), and that his verbal skills were more severely delayed than his abilities to perform perceptual motor tasks.

Visual and hearing exams were requested, and upon completion, indicated no problems.

Intervention

Bobby was admitted to the Perceptual-Motor Clinic in March of 1975. The primary objectives of his program were to promote normal reflex de-velopment, stimulate vestibular functioning, and facilitate tactile percep-tion. The reflex and vestibular activities were selected to help the child overcome his clumsiness; the tactile perception activities were designed to eliminate the tactile defensive behavior Bobby demonstrated. Examples of activities used to facilitate development in each of these areas can be found in the lesson plans at the end of this chapter.

By the end of April, 1975, some progress was seen in his overall behav-ior. Attention span remained low on most tasks; signs of frustration and task avoidance were frequent on tasks requiring any degree of concentration. Eye contact and visual fixation were inconsistent; sometimes Bobby would look at and follow an object, sometimes not. He remained uncommunicative, but did begin to demonstrate some variations in mood and facial expression. Although he continued to withdraw from contact initiated by others, he was beginning to reach out and touch some individuals. He did not participate in clinic during thet summer of 1975.

In September, 1975, Bobby began his first full semester (three months) in therapy. During this time, his tolerance for gross tactile stimulation in game activities improved dramatically but he remained sensitive to light touch (particularly to his back, shoulders, neck, and head). Auditory attention improved, once initial attention to directions could be established. Although he would auditorily attend to directions, he still avoided visually fixating on the individual giving the instructions. Attempts to engage Bobby in fine motor or quiet tasks remained difficult to accomplish, daily relaxation, tension was noted in his arms; other body parts were continuously moving. Overall activity level was markedly decreased, except when touched or excited.

At the completion of his next four-month clinic ssesion Bobby demonstrated very definite and observable improvements. Although still somewhat tactile defensive, he was beginning to positively respond to strong tactile praise, seemed to enjoy whole body tactile stimulation, and would seek opportunities to touch others; he would voluntarily sit on the therapist's lap and hug or pat the therapist on his own. Ability to perceive touch improved from awareness of single stimulation to knowledge and ability to identify where he had been touched by two stimuli applied simultaneously. Visual distractibility remain high, with constant eye shifting, unless Bobby was faced with an object of extreme interest. When required to visually pursue a moving object, his head would move, rather than just the eyes. Auditory attention improved to the point of his being able to carry out a sequence of three directions on a fairly consistent basis. Inactivity during relaxation sessions increased in terms of the length of time he was able to stay quiet and partially still (see Figure 1). The biggest improvement during this time, was the decrease in non-purposeful movement and avoidance of touch. Verbalization and communication of needs increased markedly.

By the completion of his third full semester in Clinic, Bobby was becoming a very affectionate child. He responded positively to tactile praise and stimulation, would initiate touch, and could accept being touched, as long as he could see it coming. Visual pursuit of objects was still a major problem, but Bobby was not as easily distracted by environmental sights and sounds as he had been initially. Eye-to-eye contact markedly improved over the semester and he was now able to look directly at someone while they were talking with him. Nystagmus reactions to vestibular stimulation were easily elicited and static and dynamic balance ability increased, along with control of deliberate body movement pattern. Relaxation at the end of each daily session was becoming reinforcing to him. He could contract and relax muscles over his entire body on command. Ability to express himself verbally and emotionally reached a new high. He would come into Clinic and express frustration at not being able to perform skills as well as the other children in his class at school.

During the spring and summer sessions of his fourth semester (four months) Bobby became a very eager and enthusiastic worker. Auditorily, he was aware of environmental sounds, but was not distracted by them. Although visual fixation still presented a problem in fine motor/manipulative tasks, he was able to track (binocular and monocular) moving objects horizontally and vertically in front of the face but would lose the target on diagonal movements. Relaxation continued to improve, particularly in the legs, and it was noted that Bobby relaxed better when being touched by the therapist; he now accepted touch easily and seemed reassured and calmed by it. Tactile praise became highly reinforcing and served as a tremendous motivator to the boy.

Signs of visual distress (wide eye tracking, excessive blinking, and watering of the eyes) prompted the recommendation of an additional visual examination. The examination results indicated equal use of both eyes, smooth and equal convergent/divergent movements, good depth perception, visual acuity of 20/20 in the left eye and 20/25 in the right eye, a high level of visual distractibility, and a short visual attention span. No prescription was recommended.

By December of 1977, nystagmus was easily elicited, regardless of the body position during vestibular stimulation activities. Body control during balance tasks had become smoother and more efficient. Jumping, skipping, and other bilateral integration activities were beginning to be demonstrated. Visual attention to fine motor tasks improved to the point where Bobby could look at and color a complete page in a primary level coloring book without distractions. Between activities, rather than running aimlessly around the room, Bobby would stay with his therapist and assist in getting out and returning materials and equipment. He had finally conquered his restlessness during relaxation period and could remain totally quiet for the full five minutes.

Between April, 1975 and December, 1977, Bobby spent the equivalent of 24 months in actual therapy. The sessions were 30 minutes in length for three or four days per week. The last five minutes of every session were spent in conscious relaxation attempts. Data on the amount of time the child could remain motionless were taken during those five minute periods.

The following figure charts Bobby's improvement in ability to relax completely from the time he began in Clinic until December, 1977.

Bobby is continuing Clinic and will remain doing so as long as he performs below expectations for his age level. His progress over the last few years has been slow but consistent, and improvements in his behavior at school have been reported by his classroom teachers.

When he entered first grade last year, he was placed in a school with very high academic standards and limited structure. His classroom teacher repeatedly reported that Bobby was out of his seat and off task for the majority of the time. In her opinion, he could not follow verbal directions, she could not understand his verbalizations, and he failed to interact

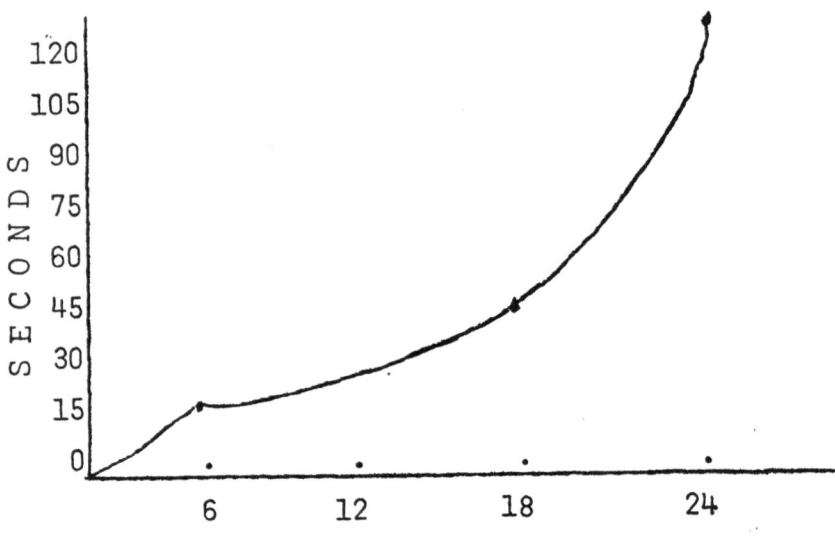

MONTHS IN THERAPY

Fig. 1. Bobby's progression in ability to remain perfectly motionless from time of entry into Clinic until December 15, 1977.

with other children. The teacher wanted him placed in a special class for retarded children.

When the school began suggesting he be retained in first grade for another year, his parents finally agreed to permit the school psychologist to test Bobby. He was found to have normal intelligence, but did qualify for Learning Disability Resource Room assistance. He was transferred to a school with a program designed to help learning disabled children, and began receiving special assistance at the beginning of the second grade.

His present teacher reports that, during this year, Bobby's speech has greatly improved, he can and will remain seated at his desk, and he stays on task nearly as long as his classmates. He has to be prompted to begin any series of academic tasks, but proceeds on his own once he begins. He is demonstrating good interaction with his peers on the playground and participating in group activities.

Conclusion

The changes in his behavior from one year to the next no doubt reflect the difference in types of school structures, the special academic programing being arranged for Bobby, and his accumulated perceptual-motor therapy experiences. It will be interesting to continue to work with this child and observe whether his progress remains consistent, or if his behavior will fluctuate as he changes teachers each year.

In this case of tactile defensiveness, the combination of tactile stimulation and conscious relaxation seemed to reduce the child's hyperactivity and influence his ability to remain motionless at will. Intervention designed to reduce abnormal reflexes and stimulate vestibular functioning also proved effective. It is most obvious that Bobby is a long way from demonstrating normative standard perceptual-motor performances; however, now that the basic sensory-input systems are functioning efficiently, Bobby will most likely progress in fine and gross motor skills. That is, he has the basic information on which to build higher level functions, and there is no reason to expect him to do otherwise.

References

AYRES, A. J. *Sensory Integration and Learning Disorders*. Los Angeles: Western Psychological Services, 1974.

AYRES, A. J. *Southern California Sensory Integration Tests*. Los Angeles: Western Psychological Services, 1972.

BOBATH, K. and BOBATH, B. A facilitation of normal postural reactions and movements in the treatment of cerebral palsy. *Physiotherapy*. 1964, 50:246-262.

DE QUIROS, J. B. and SCHRAGER, O. L. *Neuropsychological Fundamentals in Learning Disabilities.* San Rafael: Academic Therapy Publications, 1978.

FROSTIG, M. and HORNE, D. *The Frostig Program for the Development of Visual Perception.* Chicago: Follet, 1964.

GETMAN, G. N., KANE, E. R., and McKEE, G. W. *Developing Learning Readiness: A Visual-Motor Tactile Skills Program.* Manchester, Mo.: Webster Division, McGraw-Hill, 1968.

KEPHART, N. C. *The Brain-Injured Child in the Classroom.* Chicago: National Society for Crippled Children and Adults, 1963.

STOCKMEYER, S. A. *The Interpretation of the Approach of Rood to the Treatment of Neuromuscular Dysfunction. Amer. J. Physical Med.* 1967, 46:900-956.

Examples of Bobby's Lesson Plans

Individual therapy programs are designed for each child on the basis of his/her evaluation results. Developmentally sequenced daily lesson plans are written weekly. The child's reactions to the lessons are recorded daily and summarized at the end of each week to determine progress or lack thereof.

Each child is criterion tested at the end of every semester in the areas of weakness.

Some examples of Bobby's daily lesson plans, weekly evaluations, and criterion test results follow.

Monday, September 15, 1975 (first day of first full semester)

Let Bobby pick some activities today, but don't allow him to run aimlessly around the room. Try to get him to talk to you and look at you while doing so. Note the types of activities or games he chooses and how long he sticks to them.

Evaluation:

Bobby didn't really choose any constructive activity, with the exception of crawling on the high balance beam. The rest of the time, he chose to run up and down the ramp. I, therefore, convinced him to play train with the scooter. Later, we tossed beanbags through the large plastic block. We worked on tossing over, in, through, and around the block. We finished with riding a scooterboard down the ramp and picking up a beanbag as we went by. He talked but it was quite difficult to understand his verbalizations.

Tuesday, September 16, 1975

1. *Tactile stimulation*. Pillow fight with Bobby. Note his aggressiveness or lack of it and his attention to the activity. What is his reaction to being hit? Will he stay within the (floor) boundaries set?
2. *Vestibular stimulation*. Put Bobby prone in the suspended tire with a pillow under his abdomen. Spin slowly at first to see how he tolerates this activity. Spin faster only if there are no objections on his part. Spin in both directions and check for nystagmus after each. Repeat several times.
3. *Dynamic balance*. Work solely on the low beam, concentrating on forward and backward movements. Try to keep Bobby's attention on you. He is the only child scheduled in this time slot. Hopefully, the lack of distraction by others will help him concentrate more fully on you.
4. *Eye-hand coordination*. Again, we need to gain the attention of this child before we are going to make any progress with him. Work on throwing and catching a 14″ soft rubber ball from a distance of about three or four feet. Try to get him to watch the ball as it is being thrown to him, and to watch you when he is throwing the ball back.
5. *Relaxation*. If you can get him down on the mat and halfway still and quiet, you'll be very successful. If you want him to try stretching and releasing, you will probably have to demonstrate for him.

Wednesday, September 17, 1975

1. *Tactile*. Try the trapping games with Bobby. Be sure he fully understands the directions before he begins; make him look at you while you explain. Trap him a few times using the canvas cloth and then let him trap you. Observe the following—does he avoid being trapped? If trapped, will he struggle to keep moving along the mat? Does he follow the directions given?
2. *Vestibular*. Try the metal barrel today. See if you can get him all the way back in the barrel and braced so he won't roll around inside (you may have to put a few pillows in to help brace him. Spin to the right and then check for nystagmus; spin to the left and recheck.
3. *Dynamic balance*. Repeat the work you did yesterday on the low balance beam. Note any improvements, and whether he remembered anything you taught him the day before.

4. *Free choice activity.* Let's use a weekly free choice for Bobby and see
   if he will eventually become more selective in his choices. Once he picks
   something for free choice, he must stick with it until relaxation time.
   Note what he picks and how he performs.
5. *Relaxation.* Continue from yesterday.

Evaluation for First Week:

1. *Tactile stimulation.* Seems more fearful than sensitive to touch. He
   appeared to be afraid of what to expect, but did not demonstrate
   sensitivity to the touch (hit) of the pillows or being 'trapped' in the
   canvas.
2. *Vestibular stimulation.* Demonstrated some nystagmus after spinnings,
   but objected to the spinning, so I usually got only one direction of good
   spin.
3. *Dynamic balance.* Overall, his balance is poor. Forward movement on
   the low beam is manageable with assistance, but the backward movement is uncontrollable.
4. *Eye-hand coordination.* He does not watch any object thrown to him.
   When receiving, he waits for the ball and traps it against his chest,
   rather than reaching out for it.
5. *Relaxation.* Cannot consciously relax. He twitches and fidgets most all
   the time. He won't allow me to passively move his arms and legs. Instead, he locks his joints and stiffens his limbs. At one point, he held
   his fingers still for 15 seconds.

NOTE:

> During the first semester, tactile activities were gradually added to in-
> clude brushing various textured objects (brushes, stiff netting, teflon
> scratch pads, sponges) over all parts of his body except his lower torso,
> gentle boxing matches with light boxing gloves, trapping games with a
> large coarse net, and rolling down a mat placed on a ramp. Other
> activities were included to facilitate reflex development, improve visual
> tracking ability, and practice fine motor tasks. During most gross motor
> activities Bobby wore wrist and ankle weights to stimulate kinesthetic
> awareness.

During 1976, Bobby's time in Clinic was increased to four days a week
during spring, summer, and fall. The primary objectives were: continue to
facilitate reflex development, balance, tactile discrimination, kinesthetic
awareness, visual pursuit ability, spatial relations, and coordination.

Monday, October 4, 1976

1. *Kinesthetic awareness.* Have Bobby wear ankle weights (1½ lbs.) today and 'run" up and down the chairs.
2. *Dynamic balance.* Have Bobby hop through eight tires laid end to end on the floor. Have him hop on one foot, both feet, and turn at the end of the course and return. Note his ability to maintain his balance.
3. *Tactile stimulation.* Have a pillow fight on the mat. Note his aggressiveness and protective reactions.
4. *Vestibular stimulation.* Put Bobby in the hanging net and spin him in both directions. Check for nystagmus.
5. *Foot-eye coordination.* Have Bobby stand in front of a bowling pin. He must prevent it from being hit with a soft rubber ball you throw at it. He may use only his feet to deflect the ball. How accurately does he contact the ball?
6. *Relaxation.* Have Bobby lie on the tilt table with a blindfold on. Note his tolerance for the blindfold and his ability to lie still.

Tuesday, October 5, 1976.

1. *Kinesthetic awareness.* Have Bobby wear the angle weights (1½ lbs.) during all his activities today.
2. *Dynamic balance.* Work on Bobby's walking gait by having him walk on a straight line on the floor. If he tends to pull his knees inward, make note. Emphasize heel to toe walking.
3. *Vestibular stimulation.* Work on mats doing tumbling activities such as somersaults, egg rolls and log rolls. Check for nystagmus.
4. *Kinesthetic awareness.* Have a tug of war with Bobby and you kneeling. Tell Bobby to keep his head up.
5. *Fine motor.* Work on shoe lacing and tying. Make sure to tell Bobby to make his loop close to the shoe.
6. *Relaxation.* Give Bobby a back rub.

Wednesday, October 6, 1976.

1. *Leg strength and kinesthetic awareness.* Have Bobby wear the ankle weights (1½ lbs.) throughout his activities today.
2. *Dynamic balance.* Work on the low balance beam going forward, backward, and sideways. Make sure that Bobby keeps his head up and does not hurry.

3. *Vestibular stimulation.* Spin Bobby around in the desk chair. Check for nystagmus.
4. *Fine motor.* Have Bobby use grippers (tweezers) to pick up pieces of material. Time him. Then work on tying shoeslaces.
5. *Tactile stimulation.* Play dodgeball with the other therapists and their children. Note his aggressiveness and protective reactions.
6. *Relaxation.* Have Bobby choose a place where he wants to relax.

Thursday, October 7, 1976

1. *Leg strength and kinesthetic awareness.* Have Bobby wear the ankle weights (1½ lbs.) during his activities today.
2. *Kinesthetic awareness.* Have Bobby lie supine on a towel and pull himself along the floor using a rope.
3. *Dynamic balance.* Jump rope on the trampoline today. Jump forward and backward.
4. *Body image.* Have Bobby touch various parts of your body and you will name them. Make a mistake every once and awhile and see if he can catch the error.
5. *Free choice.*
6. *Relaxation.* Relax on the trampoline, emphasizing tightening and relaxing of muscles.

NOTE:

By December, 1976 two trace primitive reflexes were still evident and two equilibrium reflexes were not yet consistently demonstrated. Bobby was seeking tactile experiences (hugging), he could balance on one foot with eyes open (17 seconds) and closed (6½ seconds), he could hop, walk a high balance beam without assistance, contract and relax all his limbs at will during relaxation, and lie still for 45 seconds. His monocular and binocular tracking had improved but he preferred not to maintain eye-to-eye contact when talking to someone.

Evaluation for Week of October 4-7, 1976:

1. *Vestibular stimulation.* Bobby will demonstrate a strong nystagmus if he is spun for at least two minutes. He doesn't like to be spun and becomes uneasy if we persist for more than two minutes.
2. *Kinesthetic awareness.* He seems to be unaware that he is wearing ankle weights. They don't appear to bother him at all.

3. *Tactile stimulation.* Bobby does not seem to mind being hit, in fact, this week he wouldn't even attempt to avoid being hit. He just giggled throughout the pillow fight, and let me hit him all over with the pillow.
4. *Fine motor.* It's difficult to get Bobby to concentrate on fine motor tasks. His tendency is to look around rather than attend to the task. He wore boots all week, so we couldn't practice lacing and tying his own shoes.
5. *Balance.* His jumping and hopping still need lots of work. One of the problems is that his extensor thrust reflex dominates so that he doesn't bend at the knee and hip.
6. *Relaxation.* Bobby is tense when placed in a supine position; however, he relaxes much better when he lays face down. Perhaps his tonic labyrinthine supine reflex is contributing to his body extension.

During 1977, Bobby continued to demonstrate improvement in all areas in which we were working. The following lesson plans and evaluation reflect this growth.

Monday, November 21, 1977

1. *Reflex testing.* Test for the Landau, positive supporting reactions, body righting acting on the body, and associated reactions.
2. *Vestibular stimulation.* Place a pillow in the bottom of the hanging tire and have Bobby lay inside in a prone position. Spin the tire in both left and right directions. Note duration of spin and evidence of nystagmus. Does he express dizziness?
3. *Dynamic balance.* Have Bobby jump on the large trampoline. Work on the use of arms for height and on the knee drop. Observe for leg flexion on bounces and transition from flexion to extension during the knee drops. Stress correct posture and use of head for balance. Can he stay in one spot while bouncing?
4. *Foot control.* Walk the length of the blue mat with Bobby doing a "Penguin walk" (toes out, short waddle steps) and an "Ostrich walk" (large floppy toe-heel steps out to the side.) Stress outward position of the feet. Can he imitate these walks? Note foot position, body compensation, and use of head and arms for balance.
5. *Relaxation.* Relax in a prone position over a rolled up mat. Check for flexor tone in arms, legs, hips and neck.

Tuesday, November 22, 1977

1. *Foot control.* On the blue mats sit facing each other with legs straight. Have Bobby point his toes toward your toes and hold for four seconds. Note foot position. Discourage any inward turn of the feet and body compensation. Make sure he sits up straight and is not leaning back. Is he more efficient with either one foot or the other?
2. *Eye-hand coordination.* Play a game of catch with Bobby. Use a soft rubber utility ball and stand about six feet apart. Stress arm leg opposition and concentration on the target when throwing. Discourage trapping when catching. Note accuracy and control of throws, posture and balance after throwing, and visual attentiveness.
3. *Static balance.* Have Bobby balance a bean bag on his head while trying to maintain his balance in quadriped, triped, biped, and monoped positions. Check his balancing ability both with eyes open and closed. Check for 20 seconds in each position with eyes open and 15 seconds with eyes closed. Note use of head and arms for balance.
4. *Tactile awareness.* Move to a quiet corner of the room and have Bobby lie down in a supine position on a mat. Ask him to close his eyes and point to where you touch him. Use single and dual points of stimulation. Note correct and incorrect responses. Does he identify both areas of double stimulation?
5. *Relaxation.* Relax in supine position on mat. Rotate his legs outward from the hips so that his toes point out away from his body. Maintain this position for 40 seconds. During this time work on release of extensor tone in arms by gently shaking his arms. Note body compensation for foot position and any evidence of release of flexor tone in the arms.

Monday, November 28, 1977

1. *Reflex testing.* Test status of the following reflexes: tonic labyrthine supine and prone and symmetrical tonic neck 1 and 2.
2. *Dynamic balance.* Play a game of hopscotch with Bobby. Note his form and accuracy while hopping. Does he prefer either foot while hopping? When coming down on both feet, do they land simultaneously? Note the use of head and arms, and overall body position. Stress head up. Note foot placement.
3. *Equilibrium reactions.* Have Bobby assume a quadriped position on the tilt table. Tilt the table suddenly from side to side. Note his ability to right his head and thorax. Check for any initiation of equilibrium and

protective reactions. Stress head up and don't let him spread his arms and legs out of 90-degree angles from his body.

4. *Spatial relations.* Play follow-the-leader on the climbing equipment, taking turns being the leader. Have Bobby wear weights (1½ lbs.) on both his wrists and his ankles. Note hand and foot placement in all directions and his ability to move downward and backward. Does he move more slowly and/or less confidently in certain directions?

5. *Relaxation.* Relax on an eight-inch-wide board in supine position. Bend his knees and place his feet flat on the board with knees together. Have him maintain position for 35 seconds. Note body compensation for leg and feet positioning, and muscle tone in arms. How long can he remain perfectly still without fidgeting?

Thursday, November 29, 1977

1. *Foot control.* Have Bobby stand in a square on the floor. Place five marbles on his right side. Have him pick up the marbles one at a time with his toes and drop them in a can on that same time. Make sure he keeps his body straight and turns just his legs. Note use of head and arms, and foot position.

2. *Spatial relations.* Set up an obstacle course using the interlocking squares, bowling pins, and tires. Have Bobby go through it twice with his eyes open, then blindfold him and give him directions through it. Have him attempt this twice taking off the blindfold between trials to allow him to re-orient himslef. Note body maneuveribility, hesitation to commands, and wrong moves. Have Bobby wear ankle weights during this task.

3. *Eye-hand coordination.* Set a target on the wall at Bobby's chest height. Stress arm/leg opposition when throwing. See if he can do this in one movement (as opposed to stepping and then throwing). Note eye contact with target and distractibility. How does visual attentiveness effect his accuracy? Note accuracy after 10 throws.

4. *Fine motor.* Have Bobby color a picture in a coloring book. Stress slowness and accuracy. Can he stay within the lines? Note how he holds and controls the crayons and distance of his head from the page. Any tilt of head? Facial overflow?

5. *Relaxation.* Let Bobby choose a place to relax today. Position his supine and work on release of tension in upper and lower extremities. Any decrease in extensor tone in arms and legs?

Evaluation for weeks of November 21 and 28, 1977

1. *Reflex testing.* Landau, positive supporting, tonic labyrinthine prone, symmetrical tonic neck 1 and 2 have been inhibited. During body righting acting on the body there is occasional flexion of the right knee when he turns right. During tonic labyrinthine supine tension is still demonstrated in the left side. Associated reactions are present in right arm and legs when he squeezes a ball with his left hand.
2. *Vestibular.* Nystagmus was demonstrated for seven seconds after spinning to the right for 15 seconds; the same was elicited after turning left for 15 seconds. Also, he said he felt dizzy.
3. *Dynamic balance.* Efficient use of arms to gain height during trampoline jumping. Completed four knee-drops to standing position in a row. Tendency to droop head unless reminded to keep it up. Some trouble staying in center of trampoline while jumping.
4. *Foot control.* Cannot place heels together with toes pointed out, but he did not toe in. He is better able to position the right foot than the left. Can point toes and hold for five seconds.
5. *Relaxation.* Supine position. Slight evidence of extensor tone in legs (but it's getting better!) and some increased tension in left arm. Right arm is very relaxed. Child can lie still without fidgeting for 1 minute, 45 seconds.
6. *Eye-hand coordination.* Throwing action consists of separate stepping and throwing moves. He needs constant encouragement to watch the target while throwing, but will do it when reminded. Consistently catches ball in his hands now, rather than trapping it in his arms.
7. *Tactile Awareness.* Identified all single and double stimulation points accurately.
8. *Spatial relations.* Moved more slowly and with better control when blindfolded than without his eyes covered. Climbed all around the equipment showing no hesitation in any direction (even went down backward with little looking behind).
9. *Fine motor.* Bobby kept changing grips on his crayon and showed little control. He leaves a lot of the picture blank and shows facial overflow when coloring. He tries to stay in the lines, but does it by filling in the picture close to the lines.

CASE STUDY #14. PERCEPTUAL-MOTOR TRAINING WITH A SIX-YEAR-OLD GIRL

Jean Pypher

Current Problem

At age six, Rene was referred to the Perceptual-Motor Clinic by her family's physician, because he was concerned about her poor hand-foot-eye coordination. At the time of her referral, she had already been receiving gross motor training, for four months, three times weekly, from a learning disability teacher. Although her parents reported her to be "well adjusted in her mind, but slow in coordination," her kindergarten teacher indicated that she did not seem able to understand or follow directions. The teacher checked the following behaviors as characteristic of Rene: overactive, difficulty in concentrating, fearful, and clumsy.

Background Information

Both the parents and the family physician reported a normal pregnancy and birth. Rene was the first born of two children; her sister was born four years later. After a 30-hour "easy" labor, during which a general anesthesia was used, Rene was born weighing 7 lbs. 8½ oz. and was 21 inches in length.

Her parents reported that she sat without support at six months of age, and crawled at eight months, but did not walk without assistance until she was 18 months old. She could dress herself by the age of four, button clothes and zip zippers by the age of five, and lace shoes and buckle belts when she was six-year-old; she could not yet tie bows. Her speech development was reported as normal.

Rene was six-years, four-months old when she was tested. The evaluator described her as extremely active, inattentive, and very verbal, with cooperation ranging from fair to poor. Rene did not seem distracted by outside noises, but it was necessary for us to frequently repeat directions. She demonstrated four primitive reflexes and lacked eight equilibrium reactions. During tactile tests, she located all single points of stimuli to the body, but did not report being touched on the hands during all double-point stimulation to hands and cheeks. She withdrew from all touches and pats of praise from the evaluator. Rene was very distractable during our visual perception tests—her monocular and binocular visual tracking were very jerky and she often turned her head, rather than her eyes, as she tracked. The optometrist who tested her indicated that the internal and external examinations were unremarkable, but the subjective tests yielded poor results, because Rene was "fidgety" throughout the testing.

All static and dynamic balance tasks she attempted were reportedly extremely poor. She could not maintain her balance during single hops, nor could she sustain a continuous hopping pattern. She tended to run flatfooted with a straight posture and little "leaping" movements. Rene could not locate her ankles or hips when asked to; she tended to over- and under-estimate space requirements when moving around objects; her eye-hand and foot-eye coordination were below expectations for her chronological age. Fine motor demands frustrated both Rene and her evaluator. Rene could not seem to understand the simplest motor planning tasks, motor speed of the hands was slower than normal for a four-year-old child, and she held her pencil in a fist-like grip. During reproduction of forms, she continually turned the paper and segmented the drawings; some of the reproductions were unidentifiable. Her self drawing lacked legs, feet, toes, hands, hair, and ears; she scribbled all over the drawing after completing it.

Because Rene's family lived several miles from where the clinic was located, she did not begin a program until approximately 12 months after testing. At the end of the spring during which she was originally tested, her family moved to within a few miles of the clinic. However, her parents did not contact the clinic until October and then, only because of the urging of the classroom teacher, they called the clinic about the possibility of retesting Rene's development. At that time, Rene was six-years, 11-months old. She was enrolled in the first grade at an "open" school, where a loosely structured, learned environment was employed. Her teacher was concerned because it seemed impossible to teach the child.

Rene was retested in October, 1976. The testing took place on two different days, one day apart. The evaluator did not see the results of Rene's first test until after her reevaluation was completed.

The results of the second test were as follows: Rene demonstrated four primitive reflexes and lacked six equilibrium reactions (an improvement of two equilibrium reflexes over her first test results). Rene did not acknowledge being touched on the right hand during the single-point tactile stimulation test. During simultaneous double-point stimulation, she failed to identify one point during each of the six tests, however, there was no discernible pattern to her errors. At that time, she responded to tactile praise with a smile, and there was no indication of discomfort while she was seated. During the visual pursuit tests, her eye patterns were extremely jerky and she tended to try to follow the target by moving her entire head rather than just her eyes. In addition, her eyes jerked markedly when she attempted to visually pursue a target passing through the midline in front of her body (i.e., her eyes "jumped" as they attempted to follow a target passing in front of her nose from left to right and vice versa).

Rene seemed to have difficulty understanding auditory instructions, and was easily distracted by other noises in the room. It was necessary to repeat directions numerous times throughout the testing.

All static and dynamic balance test results were approximately three years below normal expectations for Rene's age. She could not hop on her right foot without touching the floor with her free foot, but was able to maintain her balance throughout forward movement on the low balance beam. She tended to toe-out and demonstrated tension overflow in her hands and mouth while running. She could not maintain her balance during backward walking patterns on the floor and low balance beam.

Rene identified all body parts, but showed no consistent knowledge of left and right. There was hesitancy and inaccuracy during all attempts to imitate arm movement patterns. Overflow movement to other limbs was demonstrated during all arm and leg movements in the 'angels-in-the-snow" test item.

Rene continued to grip writing implements with her fist. Her printing was barely recognizable, with poor spacing of letters and words. Reproductions of geometric forms were extremely inaccurate, with no discernible organization on the page. She appeared frustrated during all fine motor tasks; sighing, looking at the examiner, and demonstrating tension in her face. Rene's self drawing lacked ears, a mouth, neck, shoulders, waist, elbows, fingers, knees, feet, and toes; however, this time she did not scribble over the drawing after completing it. Her combined gross and fine motor test score was below the first percentile norm for her age.

We concluded that the child demonstrated sensory input delay in the areas of reflex, tactile, vestibular, visual, and kinesthetic development. It was recommended that a concentrated perceptual motor program to stimulate sensory input systems be implemented immediately.

Intervention

The results of Rene's second evaluation were discussed with her parents on November 1, 1976. They seemed somewhat concerned about the report, but continually stated that they didn't notice any problems at home. They didn't think they could arrange transportation to the clinic, but did agree to permit us to send the test results to her teacher with some suggested activities for the child to participate in at school.

Rene's teacher did try to incorporate our suggestions, but because she was unsuccessful in all of her attempts to teach the child through any sensory modality, the school urged the parents to transfer Rene to a more structured school setting and enroll her in the Perceptual-Motor Clinic as soon as possible.

In January, 1977, Rene was transferred to a different school. She began to come to the clinic three days a week, beginning on February 28. The objectives for her first semester with us were to promote tolerance to gross tactile stimulation, to elicit eye nystagmus following spinning activities, to inhibit flexor tone in the legs while in a prone position, and to facilitate relaxation. Activities included pillow fights, brushing with rough textures, massage, and wrestling for tactile stimulation; spinning, rolling, and vigorous turning for vestibular stimulation (to elicit nystagmus); concentrated scooter-board work in a prone position to override the flexor tone in the legs; and autogenic relaxation techniques.

At the end of the first two-month semester in clinic, it was reported that Rene was responding positively to manipulation, brushing, and strong massage administered by the therapist, and was becoming aggressive and persistent when initiating her own brushing. After vigorous spinning (which she thoroughly enjoyed), duration and strength of nystagmus was minimal; she never reported feeling dizzy. Inhibition of flexor tone in the legs was becoming evident, but she was still constantly moving around during the five-minute relaxation period at the end of each daily session. She would not respond to greetings when arriving at the clinic, nor would she interact with other children. When faced with an activity that she did not enjoy or she perceived as difficult, she would cross her arms and say "no," or run to another area of the room and initiate some activity other than that requested.

In a staffing session at Rene's school, the school psychologist reported that, although observation indicated otherwise, cognitive test results placed the child in the borderline-retardation range. The Learning Disability Resource teacher indicated that Rene could not order or sequence information provided auditorally or visually. Rene could identify words, but could not read, because her eyes "jumped" all over the page. Because of her height (she is a very tall child) and her age (7½) she was promoted to second grade, and her parents were urged to continue sending her to the Perceptual-Motor Clinic. Although recommended, the parents did not enroll her in summer clinic.

Rene returned to the clinic in the fall of 1977. Activities to promote inhibition of tonic labyrinthine reflexes in the prone and supine positions, vestibular functioning, kinesthetic awareness, dynamic balance, and conscious relaxation were included in her weekly lessons.

A complete battery of tests administered at the end of that semester revealed four traces of primitive reflexes and some protective movements during all equilibrium reflex tests. All single points of stimulation were accurately identified, but simultaneously applied double-point stimulation to the hands and cheeks was perceived only on the cheeks. Rene was able to visually pursue all moving targets smoothly, except those following a diagonal path. During diagonal pursuit, her eyes still moved in a somewhat jerky pattern. She still had difficulty remembering directions and was easily distracted by other sounds in the room. Nystagmus was strong but persisted for only half of the desired duration. Gross-motor-skill efficiency had improved; however, frustration was still demonstrated during fine motor tasks. For the first time, it was reported that Rene could put her own shoes and socks on. She was very cooperative, once her attention was gained. Rene was beginning to permit her therapist to passively flex and extend her limbs during relaxation time, but remaining absolutely still without fidgeting or talking, escaped her. She continued in clinic.

Finally, a definite breakthrough began to occur during the spring of 1978. Activities to promote vestibular stimulation, dynamic balance, laterality, arm and leg strength, primitive reflex inhibition, and conscious relaxation were concentrated on. Because her equilibrium reactions had improved dramatically during the previous fall 1977, we were able to include more trampoline jumping exercises without fear of Rene's losing her balance and possibly falling. In our situation, trampoline activities have proven successful in providing kinesthetic stimulation necessary to inhibit primitive reflexes and faclitate lower body strength and, hence, gross body control. As a result of improved voluntary neuromuscular control, Rene learned to execute a series of movements (seat drop, knee drop, coordination of arm and leg patterns) on the trampoline. She also learned to jump rope (on the floor), while turning the rope herself. She developed a consistent knowledge of left and right on her own body, walked the high balance beam forward with head up and eyes straight ahead, and began to lie still without fidgeting or talking during conscious relaxation. Observational data gathered during conscious relaxation that semester follows:

Her eye nystagmus after spinning still did not continue for the duration we would have preferred (20 seconds), but this was gradually improving.

In May, 1978, Rene's resource teacher reported that several gains were beginning to be evident in her academic work. Her ability to visually track consecutive lines while reading had improved tremendously. This visual

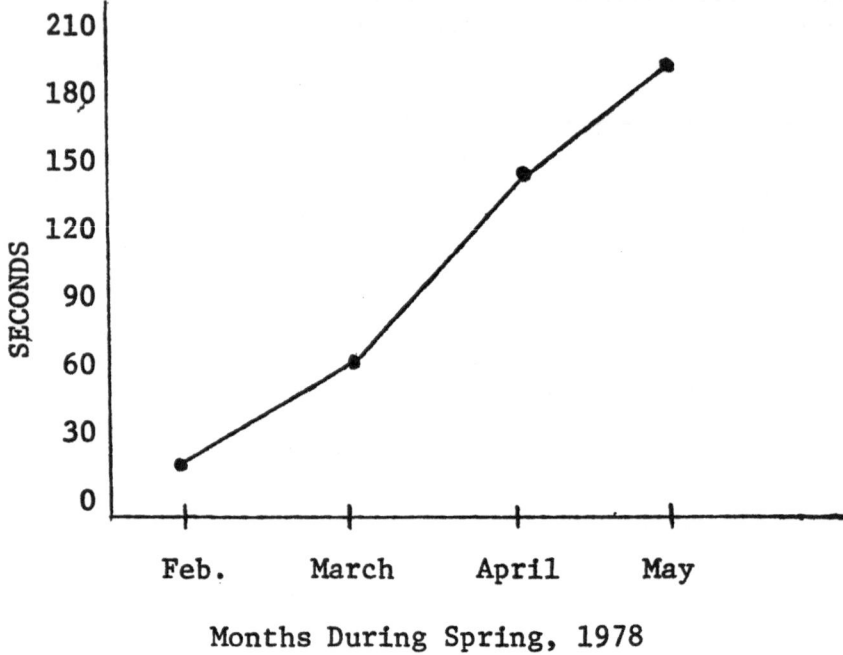

Fig. 2. Rene's progression in ability to remain perfectly motionless during five-minute relaxation periods, Spring Semester, 1978.

control resulted in increased reading comprehension. Rene was also attending to assigned tasks for longer periods of time. When faced with a new task, instead of saying "no" and walking away, she was willing to try. The biggest changes seemed to be in her improved fine motor control and ability to make friends with children her own age. Her classroom teacher, resource teacher, and clinic personnel agreed that Rene had a long way to go, but she seemed to have a healthy start.

Conclusion

Rene's case has been included here because she seems to represent the type of child who has such a large range of sensory input problems, that little if any cognitive learning seems possible. It was interesting to note, that not until the third semester of clinic intervention, did Rene begin to "get things together"—both in the clinic and the classroom. Her progress by the end of the spring semester of 1978 was very promising and, after a summer without the clinic, she continued to show gains during the fall. If she continues to gain at her present rate, she will achieve normative standard performance and be released from the perceptual-motor clinic at the end of the spring 1979 semester.

Examples of Rene's Lesson Plans

Week of March 28-31, 1977

Monday, March 28

1. *Tactile.* Rene in a prone position on a mat. Massage the neck, shoulders and back. Check for reaction to stimulation by hands in stroking, petrissage, etc. Check for tightness in muscles.
2. *Tonic labyrinthine prone.* Have Rene do a series of seal walks, where primary emphasis will be on extension of the legs. Watch for flexion of the legs and verbally correct such moves.
3. *Vestibular.* Rene will be asked to do a consecutive number of forward rolls. Observe amount of tuck she uses and forward momentum of the whole body. Note duration and strength of nystagmus.
4. *Dynamic balance.* Ask Rene to hop on one foot and then the other in a circular motion. Observe use of arms, height of hops, ability to persist without touching free foot on floor.
5. *Relaxation.* Autogenic relaxation while in a supine position. Use instructions such as "Your body is heavy against the floor," "Your arm is heavy," etc.

Tuesday, March 29

1. *Tactile.* Have Rene "rub out" an area on her body that you touch. Note the difference to intensity of touch and how she responds to it.
2. *Tonic labyrinthine prone.* Have Rene lay down prone on a scooter. In this position have her push away from the wall (using feet only) and try to project herself (on the scooter) to a bowling pin placed 20 feet from the wall. Remind her to keep her head up. Repeat several times.
3. *Vestibular stimulation.* With Rene still on the scooter in a prone position, have her take hold of one end of a six-foot rope. You hold the other end of the rope and spin her around for several seconds. Alternate

directions. Check duration of nystagmus, often turning her in each direction.

4. *Dynamic balance.* Have Rene sit on the large rubber ball that has a handle on the top. Ask her to do "kangaroo jumps" while sitting on the ball holding onto the handle. Note amount of leg extension and her ability to maintain equilibrium.

5. *Relaxation.* Rene on her back on a mat. Give instructions to her such as "Your body is warm; Your arm is becoming warm; Imagine you are rolled up in a blanket and are very warm." Note her reaction to this technique and check limbs for amount of relaxation.

Thursday, March 31

1. *Tactile.* Have a pillow fight with Rene. Emphasize hitting below the neck. Note aggressiveness and whether she attempts to protect herself or retreat. Does she keep a good grasp on the pillow?

2. *Tonic labyrinthine prone.* Have Rene lay prone on the scooter-board and descend the inclined board several times. Remind her to keep her head up and extend her limbs.

3. *Vestibular stimulation.* Put Rene in the metal barrel; have her curl up inside and brace against the sides. Spin the barrel on its side. Stop several times and check for nystagmus.

4. *Free choice.* Permit Rene to choose any activity. Note how long it takes her to make the selection, what she selects, and how well she does.

5. *Relaxation.* Rene in any position she chooses on a mat. Ask her to think about her favorite color. Watch to see if she keeps her eyes closed and if she keeps her body motionless.

Evaluation of weekly activities

1. *Tactile.* Rene identified areas that were touched during massage and seemed very relaxed around the shoulders. She enjoyed the "rub out" game and seemed to respond best to a soft touch. She laughed a lot during the pillow fight, protected herself adequately, but seemed hesitant to hit me with her pillow. She did not swing many times, but would do so when I encouraged her.

2. *Vestibular stimulation.* Minimal nystagmus was elicited during these activities. She seemed to enjoy them, but never did complain of being dizzy.

3. *Tonic labyrinthine prone.* Most of the activities were performed correctly, but she had difficulty pushing off from the wall with her feet.

It was almost as if she wasn't sure how to extend her legs vigorously to initiate the movement of the scooter.

4. *Dynamic balance.* Can hop on both feet easily, but has difficulty when hop is confined to one foot. She complained of being tired when I kept asking her to hop on one foot. Accomplished the "kangaroo hops" on the ball with vigor. Good leg extension and fairly good control of balance.
5. *Relaxation.* Always moves around during relaxation. Won't keep her eyes shut. Remained motionless for 10 seconds.

Week of October 3-6, 1977

Monday, October 3

1. *Tonic labyrinthine prone.* Lying prone on a scooter have Rene ride down the incline, and then two rows of tires that make a path straight from the incline. Watch for arm flexion.
2. *Vestibular stimulation.* Have Rene curl up in the back of a barrel that is lying on its side on the floor. Spin her 20 seconds and then check strength and duration of nystagmus. Repeat in the opposite direction.
3. *Dynamic balance.* Have Rene walk the low and high balance beam without your assistance. Have her hold a stick horizontal to her body and walk slowly forward, backward, and sideways. Watch for loss of balance and be ready to support her.
4. *Laterality.* Play "Simon Says." For example, tell her to do something with her right arm as you do it. Watch for overflow, delayed response, and distractibility.
5. *Relaxation.* Permit Rene to select one place to lay down, and then do not permit her to change places. She should not be allowed to talk. Massage her gently and check for any aversion to being touched, especially if you reprimand her for moving or talking.

Wednesday, October 5

1. *Tonic labyrinthine prone.* Have Rene lay over a barrel that is on the floor on its side. Roll the barrel slowly forward so that she must take her weight on her hands. Support her carefully. Watch for arm flexion.
2. *Vestibular stimulation.* Rene will lay on the scooter-board in a prone position. Spin her by pulling her around in circles while she holds onto the rope you are using. Check for strength and duration of nystagmus.

3. *Dynamic balance.* Play hopscotch with Rene. Watch for overflow, coordination of arms and legs while hopping and distractibility.
4. *Laterality.* Do ballet movements with Rene. Tell her to point her left or right leg and raise her right or left arm. Watch for confusion of directions, overflow, and distractibility.
5. *Relaxation.* Let Rene choose one place to lie down and do not let her move from that position. Do not permit her to talk. Massage her back. Check for aversion to being touched.

Thursday, October 6

1. *Tonic labyrinthine prone.* Rene will ride down the incline board on a scooter in a prone position. As she accelerates, have her throw a bean bag through a suspended hoop. Watch to see if she fully extends her arm after the throw.
2. *Vestibular stimulation.* Have Rene crawl into the cheesecloth tunnel, get someone to help you swing her from side to side. Check for strength and duration of nystagmus.
3. *Dynamic balance.* Using a 12-inch, soft rubber ball, play "catch in the moonwalk." Watch for loss of balance and/or any inability to remain in a standing position.
4. *Directionality.* Play "Twister" with Rene. Watch for confusion of left and right and for distractibility.
5. *Relaxation.* Have Rene choose one place to lie down and do not permit her to verbalize. Massage her. Check for aversion to touch.

Evaluation of weekly activities.

1. *Tonic labyrinthine prone.* Arm flexion is still exhibited but less than last week. She needs constant encouragement to keep her arms straight, but seems to do a better job when the activities are exciting (i.e., on the scooter-board).
2. *Vestibular.* Rene expressed displeasure of the vestibular activities. She demonstrated no nystagmus at all after vigorous spinning.
3. *Dynamic balance.* Her balance and coordination were good when she didn't have to concentrate on things, such as the rules to hopscotch. She seemed fearful of the high balance beam; she walked on it but only while holding my hand. She really enjoyed the moonwalk and did not want to get out when our time was up. She could maintain her balance while throwing, but not while catching.

4. *Laterality and directionality.* She does not know her left from her right. She was slow in reacting to left and right commands, and was obviously guessing as she responded. She was highly distracted during these activities.
5. *Relaxation.* Rene demonstrated extensor tone in her legs while on her back. When lying face down, her arms tend to flex. Verbalization was decreased from last week and she did not appear to mind being touched.

Week of April 17-20, 1978

Tuesday, April 18

1. *Vestibular stimulation.* Spin Rene once in each direction for 20 seconds. Check for strength and duration of nystagmus. Any dizziness observed or any complaints of dizziness?
2. *Dynamic balance.* Have Rene walk on a side lying barrel placed on a mat. Have her balance a bean bag on her shoulder during the activity. Is she able to keep her balance on the barrel? Does she have any difficulty walking the barrel? Does she keep her feet in the center of the barrel or do they get too far forward or behind the center? Is she able to keep the bean bag balanced on her shoulder? Does she keep her head up and make good use of her arms to help balance? How is her attentiveness?
3. *Laterality and directionality.* Have Rene stand on the low balance beam and give her commands to turn and/or walk left, right, forward, backward. Is Rene able to choose right and left correctly? Does she readily recognize any errors she makes? Is Rene able to maintain her balance on the beam and keep her concentration on the task?
4. *Strength-kinesthesis.* Have Rene lay supine on the mat under the rope. Have her pull herself into a sitting position with her hands and, if possible, on up into a standing position. Does she have enough strength to pull herself into these positions? Does she complete the task rapidly or slowly? Is it easy or a struggle? Ask her if she is tired after this activity.
5. *Relaxation.* Have Rene lay supine on the trampoline with a pillow under her head and her knees. Have her tense her entire body and then relax. Passively flex Rene's arm or legs? Is Rene able to relax fully after periods of tension? Explain to her exactly what you are looking for in relaxation (heavy and limp arms). Does she really seem to be trying?

Wednesday, April 19

1. *Vestibular stimulation.* Spin Rene in the barrel once in each direction for 20 seconds. Check strength and duration of nystagmus. Is Rene dizzy? Check for any staggering in her walk after spinning activity.
2. *Dynamic balance.* Work with Rene on jumping rope. Have her jump rope by herself. Is she able to jump at correct time or does she jump too soon or too late? Is she able to maintain good balance while jumping? Does she stay in one place when jumping or does she use a large space of the floor? Does she keep her head up? Is she concentrating?
3. *Laterality.* Play catch with the bean bags. Each of you designate which hand the other is to catch the bean bag with. Is Rene able to catch the bean bag with the hand you call or is she still confusing left and right? Note her accuracy in catching and throwing the bean bags.
4. *Strength-kinesthesis.* Have a race with Rene in the hall using different modes of locomotion. (Running, jumping, hopping.) Does Rene tire easily in this activity? Is she able to put forth good effort? Is she able to maintain good balance in jumping and hopping? Does she enjoy the activity?
5. *Relaxation.* Have Rene relax on the mat today with a pillow under her head and knees. Tell her to relax and lay perfectly still. Check for relaxation of arms and legs. Any dominant extensor tone seen in the legs? Is she fidgety?

Thursday, April 20

1. *Dynamic balance.* Have Rene jump rope on the bag trampoline. Is she able to keep her balance well on the trampoline? Any difficulty seen in jumping rope? Does she keep her head up. Is she concentrating? Does she enjoy the activity?
2. *Laterality and directionality.* Have Rene get down on all fours on the mat; give her directions of left, right, backward, and forward and have her crawl in that direction. Is she able to discriminate between the directions? Does she recognize any errors she makes?
3. *Strength-kinesthesis.* Put ankle weights on Rene and lay supine on mat with her. Raise her legs in the air and pretend to ride a bicycle. Is she able to keep her legs in the air and keep them moving? Any difficulty with this activity? Does she tire easily or complain of being tired?
4. *Free choice.* Let Rene choose an activity to do for approximately five minutes. Note her choice of activity and her performance in the activity.

Does she attend to the task? Is it an activity where you can both participate, or just Rene only?

5. *Relaxation.* Have Rene relax on the trampoline and record the time she remains still and doesn't talk. Stress to her the importance of not talking and keeping her eyes closed.

Evaluation of weekly activities.

1. *Vestibular.* Nystagmus duration is still not one-half the spinning time, but in barrel nystagmus lasted about nine seconds and was fairly strong. No signs of dizziness seen; no staggering in walk.
2. *Dynamic balance.* Balance is very good when jumping rope but we are still having problems walking on the barrel. She knows what she needs to do but can't execute movements all the time. Head position is usually good, but arms are used minimally. She doesn't seem to concentrate during the barrel walking activity.
3. *Laterality and directionality.* On activities where Rene just has to discriminate between right and left, and move in that direction, she begins to make errors frequently. She's really very inconsistent—some days her selections are perfect, other days she is way off.
4. *Strength-kinesthesis.* Rene enjoys races and shows good strength in her legs. I did notice some tiring in "bicycle" activity. She kept asking me to remove the weights.
5. *Free choice.* No hesitation in choosing this activity. Held her concentration well, showed no signs of tiring after five solid minutes of the jumping on the trampoline.
6. *Relaxation.* Rene still has a hard time achieving good relaxation especially in the arms. Thursday Rene laid perfectly still for three minutes and 20 seconds, which was fantastic. We'll keep working on better relaxation of arms and legs.

CHAPTER 6

Ecological Considerations

As discussed in the introductory chapter, the hyperactive child is not defined in isolation from a behavioral setting. The perceptions, beliefs, and expectations of persons in the environment, as well as the nature of the environment itself, have an impact on the identification and course of treatment for hyperactivity. Some environments are more accommodating, and some are considerably less flexible in their adaptation to individual differences among children.

A review of the literature reveals some interesting data related to how environment interacts with the hyperactive syndrome. What the literature seems to be saying is that each hyperactive child is different; generalizations regarding what is good for *all* hyperactive children are tenuous, and each situations needs to be examined on its own terms. The nature of the interaction of child-based variables with classroom-based variables, such as seating arrangement, content and presentation of academic program, and teacher child relationship need to be considered.

The environmental destimulation model proposed by Cruikshank and his colleagues (Cruikshank et al., 1961), is an example of attempting to match an environment to a child's capability to process sensory input. However, a number of subsequent studies questioned Cruikshank's model and the efficacy of matching hyperactive children to low-stimulation environments (Sommervill et al., 1973; Rost and Charles, 1967; Shores and Havbrich, 1969). As a generalization, the environmental destimulation model seems to lack validity. But, it may work well with a given child.

A counter position to that of Cruikshank and his co-workers views the hyperactive child as under-aroused and stimulus-seeking (Zentall, 1977; Koester, 1977). From this viewpoint, the optimum environment ought not be chaotic, but should include novelty, opportunity for the child to pursue his interests, and opportunities for physical movement. Studies by Zentall and Zentall (1976), Flynn and Rapoport (1976), and Koester (1977) supported this hypothesis. While the Zentall and Zentall study used a contrived experimental setting, the Koester and Flynn, and Rapoport studies looked at open, versus traditional classrooms. The open classrooms were found to be either as effective or more effective in reducing the hyperactivity and facilitating learning. Whether such environments actually result in a reduction of hyperactive behavior; or whether they facilitate the channelling of the child's energy into more appealing activities, thereby reducing his "nuisance value" in the room; or whether more accepting and tolerant teachers are a precondition of a more open environment, which affects the assessment of hyperactivity, is not always clear. Also, while the data presented argue a generalization, it is likely that a number of hyperactive children would escalate their hyperactivity in such high-stimulus settings.

Krippner (1975) described an environment for hyperactive children that attempted to be holistic in nature. This special school setting utilized three main program components: sensory-motor training; orthomolecular medicine; and the open classroom. The opportunities for matching the child to a curricular design seemed present, as well as the teacher attitude that these children could learn and progress developmentally. The design of the study to evaluate the efficacy of the program was weak, but did present highly favorable results.

Another interesting study was reported by Bugental et al. (1977). They examined the interaction of the child's causal attribution with two treatments, a self-control and a social (other) control procedure, and the status of either medicated or non-medicated. Self-control training occurred through a tutor working with a child to develop "talking-to-yourself" strategies. This approach to cognitive self-management was described in an earlier article by Meichenbaum and Goodman (1971). Social reinforcement occurred via the tutor's responding selectively to the child's efforts. Appropriate child behavior was praised and inappropriate behavior was ignored. The child's causal attribution was measured by a questionnaire that revealed the extent to which the child attributed success or failure in school to self or others. The findings were that the teaching of self-control worked best with children who had high scores on personal causality and/or were non-medicated. The social reinforcement procedures worked best on children with low personal causality and/or were on medication.

Once again, what worked involved a match of environmental with child-based variables, rather than one procedure that was "right" for all children. The two case studies presented in this chapter illustrate the importance of ecological considerations. The first case, by Thompson and Peterson, considers a number of child-based variables and how they interact with the developed intervention program. The second study, by DeMers and Burke, focuses on how consultation was used to modify the teacher-child relationship so as to support an effective intervention program.

References

BUGENTAL, D. B. Causal attributions of hyperactive children and motivational assumptions of two behavior-change approaches: Evidence for an interactionist position. *Child Dev.* 1977, 48:874-884.

CRUICKSHANK, W. M., BENTZEN, F. A., RATEZBURG, F., and TANNHAUSER, M. T. *A Teaching Method for Brain-Injured and Hyperactive Children.* Syracuse: Syracuse University Press, 1961.

FLYNN, N. M. and RAPOPORT, R. Hyperactivity in open and traditional classroom environments. *J. Spec. Ed.* 1976, 10:285-290.

KOESTER, L. S. Arousal and hyperactivity in open and traditional education: A test of theory. *Dissertation Abstracts.* 1977, 37:5203A-5704A.

KRIPPNER, S. An alternative to drug treatment for hyperactive children. *Acad. Ther.* 1975, 10:433-439.

MEICHENBAUM, D. and GOODMAN, J. Training impulsive children to talk to themselves: A means of developing self-control. *J. Abnorm. Psychol.* 1971, 77:115-126.

ROST, K. J. and CHARLES, D. C. Academic achievement of brain injured and hyperactive children in isolation. *Except. Child.* 1967, 34:125-126.

SHORES, R. E. and HAVBRICH, P. A. Effect of cubicles in educating emotionally disturbed children. *Except. Child.* 1969, 36:21-24.

SOMERVILL, J. W., WARNBERG, L. S., and BOST, D. E. Effects of cubicles versus increased stimulation on task performance by first-grade males perceived as distractible and nondistractible. *J. Spec. Ed.* 1970, 7:169-185.

ZENTALL, S. S. Environmental stimulation model. *Except. Child.* 1977, 43:502-510.

ZENTALL, S. S. and ZENTALL, T. R. Activity and task performance of hyperactive children as a function of environmental stimulation. *J. Consulting and Clin. Psychol.* 1976, 44:693-697.

CASE STUDY #15. AN ECOLOGICAL PERSPECTIVE OF HYPERACTIVITY IN A PRESCHOOL CHILD WITH DEVELOPMENTAL DELAY

Barbara J. Thompson and Nancy L. Peterson

Current Problem

Davey had been enrolled in a community preschool for only a short period of time when it became apparent to the staff that he was significantly behind the other children and in need of some kind of special help. Although Davey was four-years-of-age, cognitively and socially, he functioned at a level much below that of his classmates. He seemed unable to participate in the regular activities of the preschool and lacked many of the skills that the other children had mastered. His behavior in the preschool classroom resulted in his teacher's describing him as developmentally delayed and hyperactive. After just three months in the community preschool, the staff concluded that he should be referred to a special program for handicapped children. In making the referral, Davey's preschool teacher reported that he was not able to function successfully in a preschool classroom. Observational data on Davey which she recorded over a two-week period indicated that he:

(a) engaged in frequent periods of random movement around the room without any constructive participation in play activity; such episodes occurred on the average of four or five times during a 20-minute activity period;

(b) engaged in a high rate of hitting, kicking, pushing, grabbing, and shoving of classmates at a frequency of about one incident per minute during free play and unstructured activities;

(c) followed only five teacher directions without prompting during an entire two-week observation period;

(d) interrupted activities with inappropriate verbal behavior on the average of five times per 20-minute period; and

(e) engaged in constructive play or work activity for a time period that averaged only three to four minutes in length.

Davey's teacher also indicated that he required an undue amount of staff time and supervision because of his disruptive and immature behavior. Not only was he aggressive with classmates, he was destructive with materials and seldom used them for their intended purpose. His interactions with classmates were infrequent and, when they did occur, they usually were disruptive to the play of others. Consequently, the children often avoided Davey and outwardly rejected his approaches. Davey's teacher felt that he had profited little from his experiences in their preschool. She suggested that he was either retarded or emotionally disturbed and was clearly "the most hyperactive child she had ever encountered in their center."

Davey's case is quite typical of children who are referred to special programs for young handicapped or "at-risk" children. The hyperactivity evidenced by Davey is one of the most frequent symptoms that alerts teachers and parents to a potential problem. Hence, it is a frequent descriptor of very young handicapped children or of children who may be identified as "at-risk" for a potential developmental disability. While a high level of activity is quite typical of a group of very young preschoolers, it is only when such behavior appears to be excessive within a particular environmental setting that the child is labeled as hyperactive. This was true of Davey. In the regular preschool setting, Davey's behavior was quite unlike that of his more advanced peers. Compared to them, his behavior was deviant; he was hyperactive. Yet, compared to a much younger child, Davey's behavior was more typical.

An ecological perspective of Davey's behavior would suggest that such a label or diagnosis of hyperactivity, in respect to a developmentally delayed or handicapped child, may actually be a function of several factors. These factors relate to the child's developmental level, his behavioral repertoire, and to the environment in which he is expected to function. First, Davey exhibited a limited behavioral repertoire, as do many handicapped and developmentally delayed preschool-age children. He possessed few social/classroom skills that allowed him to engage in constructive play and age-appropriate activity within a group setting. With so few behavioral alternatives available to him, there was a greater probability that his high energy and activity level would manifest themselves in more random, nonconstructive, and non-purposeful movement. This in itself, gives the appearance of excessive activity—or hyperactivity. Such behavior may accelerate when a child is unable to attend to or become involved in a play activity that will hold his attention for an extended period of time. Hence, random and overactive behavior results in more of the same behaviors, unless some kind of direct or indirect intervention occurs.

A second factor which may contribute to hyperactive behavior relates to the preschool environment. The preschool setting into which a handicapped or developmentally delayed child is placed may be organized to support and encourage much higher levels of behavior than the child is capable. At the same time, it may not be supportive of the more primitive developmental behaviors that are more characteristic of the child's functioning level. Consequently, the environment may provide limited stimuli for activity appropriate to the needs of the child. If a child such as Davey is unable to match his behavior to the demands of the environment, he may be left to his own more limited and primitive means of using time. From an ecological point of view, this is a clear mismatch between the environment and the child, which is manifest partially through behaviors often label as "hyperactive." It is possible that this is an all-too-frequent occurrence with handicapped or developmentally delayed preschool children who are placed in environments that are not designed nor really adapted to them.

A third and final factor relating to the ecological perspective of Davey's behavior, is that his behavior has an impact upon his own classroom environment which, in turn, affects the quality of care delivered back to him. Davey's own behavior helped to define his own preschool environment. It helped to determine how responsive that environment was to his own social and instructional needs. In Davey's case, his preschool environment was organized around expectations for much more advanced social and cognitive behavior than he was capable of. When his behavior could not meet the demands of that environment, the reactions of the children and teachers were often negative and resulted in punitive measures or withdrawal of contact. Davey was not responsive to his environment and his environment became less responsive to him. Yet, with a limited repertoire of behavioral alternatives, Davey's problem behavior was perhaps one of his only means for interacting with and gaining attention from his environment. It is from this ecological perspective and the three factors that have been used to review Davey's behavior that the treatment approach was developed and the following case study is reported.

Background Information

Davey was born on December 20, 1972; the only child of John and Mildred, who were 32 and 28 at the time of his birth. Both parents held B.A. degrees in education and taught high school science classes. Immediately following Davey's birth, his mother resigned from her teaching position to care for her son and continued to remain in the home throughout his preschool years.

A medical history disclosed no problems during the prenatal period and no difficulties during delivery. Developmental milestones noted by Davey's mother indicated that he walked at 18 months, said single words at 24 months, and was toilet trained at 30 months. Davey's general health and physical condition were consistently reported as excellent. No clear abnormalities were noted during his early years, except that his pediatrician reported that he was somewhat behind most children in reaching developmental milestones.

Both of Davey's parents described him as an easy child to manage at home. He generally played by himself, since he was an only child, and was allowed to play freely around the house and fenced yard as he pleased. His favorite play activity involved push or pull toys. However, it was difficult to get Davey to sit and look at books or to listen to stories. Consequently, the parents typically did not pressure Davey into such activities. When Davey was three-years and ten-months old, he was enrolled in the community preschool. His parents decided he needed to be around other children, since he had few opportunities to play with others in his neighborhood and he continued to seem "slower" than children of his same age.

Intervention

Intervention from an ecological perspective focuses upon the educational or treatment environment in which behavior occurs, as well as upon the child and his interactions with that environment. Davey's difficulties seemed to be as much a function of his environment as they were a function of his own behavioral disabilities. Under a different environmental setting that was more closely aligned with his developmental and social-skill levels, his behavior might not have become so deviant and inappropriate. Consequently, the intervention approach for Davey was directed toward the creation of a better match between his learning environment and his own developmental abilities and needs. A more appropriate preschool environment was designed for Davey in his new school that provided the necessary instructional programing to help him acquire the skills he lacked. It was also designed to provide more structured opportunities for him to engage in activities that were in harmony with his performance abilities.

Davey was actually placed in the special program at the time he was four-years and two-months old. Upon his enrollment, an in-depth diagnostic evaluation was conducted over a period of two weeks in the areas of speech and language, reflex development, fine and gross motor development, preacademic skills, and social behavior. Results of this evaluation are shown in Table 1. At the same time the formal evaluations were being conducted, Davey was systematically introduced to the routines, rules, and expectations within his new classroom. As he responded to the new routines, he was

TABLE 1

Davey's* Initial Evaluation Diagnostic Results

Instrument or Assessment Tool	Scores or Results
Denver Developmental:	
Social Behavior	2 yrs, 8 mos
Language Development	4 yrs
Gross Motor	3 yrs, 8 mos
Fine Motor	3 yrs
Portage Guide to Early Education	
Developmental Checklist:	
Cognitive	2 yrs, 3 mos
Social	2 yrs, 3 mos
Motor	3 yrs, 4 mos
Self-Help	3 yrs, 4 mos
Language	3 yrs, 4 mos
Fiorentino Reflex Test:	
Spinal level	(all)—
Brainstem level	(all)—
Midbrain level	(all)+
Cortical level	(all)+
TACL (Test of Auditory Comprehension	
of Language)	3 yrs, 6 mos
Goldman Fristoe Articulation Test	
Articulation	within normal limits
Expressive Language Sample and Analysis	estimated 6 months delay

* Davey's chronological age = 4 yrs 2 mos.

quickly reinforced for his appropriate and constructive behavior. (These procedures will be described later). On the basis of the results of the in-depth evaluation, and upon teacher observations of Davey's behavior and learning during his first two weeks in this new classroom, an individual activity and instructional program was developed. The developmental assessment clearly revealed that Davey did not have the necessary behaviors to interact appropriately with peers or to meet the performance expectations of his previous preschool setting. Thorough physical, neurological, and audiological examinations gave no indication of any pathological disorder as a source or contributing factor to his difficulties.

The intervention strategy or treatment program that was implemented for Davey consisted of three major components:

(a) designing the physical environment so that it was in closer alignment with Davey's developmental level and behavioral skills;

(b) providing the necessary individual training to help Davey acquire critical developmental skills; and

(c) selecting the teaching methods and training strategies that were most appropriate for Davey.

Intervention by designing the physical environment. The physical environment was designed to increase the probability that Davey would engage in more constructive social and learning activities. The environment was also arranged to assure that Davey would experience more success and reinforcement in classroom activities by providing more opportunity for him to engage in tasks appropriate to his abilities. Specifically, the environment was structured to include the following components:

A Structured Routine of Daily Activities

Davey's daily routine was set up so that it was always the same. This allowed him to anticipate events and to perform more independently in moving from one activity to the next. For example, Davey's free playtime was always between 9:10 and 9:30. His individual 1-1 tutoring, at a corner table in the classroom, always occurred at 9:30. His small-group language activity, which occurred on the round floor rug, always occurred at 10:00.

The Establishment of Clear Physical and Verbal Cues for Initiating Transitions from One Activity to the Next

Transitions from one activity to another were paired with various stimuli; such as flickering lights, music, a special song, a move to a particular place in the room, the ringing of a bell, etc. This strategy clearly designated the ending of a given activity, provided the stimulus to move to a new activity, and gave the cue for Davey and his classmates to be ready for a new task. This procedure decreased the confusion that Davey might have had as to what he should do next, and it increased the support for him in moving smoothly from one activity to another.

The Variation of Activities According to the Amount of Attention Required, the Movement Involved in the Activity, and the Structure Provided

Davey's daily schedule was arranged so that activities requiring high levels of attending behavior and little movement were followed by less cognitively demanding, physically oriented activities. This allowed Davey to direct his energies more appropriately and to expend them in a more productive manner. Davey was able to be very physically active, yet he was also regularly engaged in activities which decreased his activity level and required quieter forms of participation. For example, free playtime was followed by 1-1 tutoring. Speech therapy was followed by outdoor playground time. Outdoor playtime was followed by a quieter language development and story time activity.

The Placement of Toys and Learning Materials in Davey's
Classroom Environment That Were Specifically
Geared to His Level of Functioning

The play and learning skills in Davey's repertoire provided the basis for the selection of toys and learning materials that were made available to him. Instructional materials which were appropriate to or adapted specifically for his needs were provided during the more structured work periods. Materials and toys were thus made more attractive and interesting to Davey. He was able to play and work with them more readily. In his previous environment, the play materials were selected for a "typical" preschool classroom and were not particularly selected with Davey's particular developmental level and instructional needs in mind.

The Inclusion of Non-Delayed or Non-Handicapped Children as
Models in Specific Instructional Activities for Davey

While children are often grouped for special instruction with classmates who have similar developmental and skill levels, Davey still needed continuous exposure to more advanced and age-appropriate behavioral models. The intervention environment in which he was placed was designed as an "integrated" classroom, which included both handicapped or developmentally delayed children and non-handicapped children. Within this classroom, Davey was frequently placed with a non-delay peer model or with a group of children containing both non-handicapped children and other delayed or handicapped children. In every case, the activity in which he was engaged was still individually planned to meet his needs, as were the activities for each of the other members of his instructional group. The models typically exhibited more appropriate forms of behavior, often elicited constructive and cooperative behavior from Davey, and often served to structure the social environment so that Davey followed along with them in responding to teacher instructions. Davey was encouraged to observe his peers and he was reinforced for imitating new and appropriate play behaviors. Models were also reinforced for exhibiting constructive behavior as well as for working and playing with Davey.

The Maintenance of a Reinforcing Environment Which Provided
Systematic Reinforcement for Following Directions and
Routines, for Engaging in Appropriate Social Interactions,
and for Maintaining Constructive Activity

The roles of teachers and aides in the classroom, as well as their movement about the classroom, were organized in a way so that they could maintain high rates of reinforcement for all children, including Davey, as desired behaviors were exhibited. Reinforcement was delivered to Davey at a very high rate during the first few weeks of attendance. He was also given frequent cues and prompts to elicit positive forms of behavior. Reinforcement was gradually phased into a variable interval and ratio schedule as his behavior became more consistent.

Intervention by providing the necessary individual training and applying teaching methods that were most appropriate for Davey. A specific intervention program was designed to help Davey gain better stimulus control over his social and interactive behavior, to diminish his excessive non-purposeful behavior, and to help build the developmental skills he so clearly lacked. An individual program plan (IEP) was developed that outlined specific goals for Davey, along with the specific treatment methods that would be used with him. Teaching methods were identified that seemed to be most likely to help Davey acquire the skills he needed in order to move progressively through the intervention program that was outlined for him. Specifically, his training program included the following components:

The Initial Pairing of Extrinsic and Primary Reinforcers
with Verbal Praise and Physical Contact

When Davey entered the special program, social contact, praise, and more typical forms of social reinforcement were not effective as reinforcers for him. Therefore, small trinkets and edibles, such as cereal and raisins were paired with praise and other social reinforcements. This was continued until Davey's behavior was stabilized and he responded positively to social forms of reinforcement.

The Gradual Expansion of Work Time on a Particular Task or Activity to Build Upon Davey's Attending Skills

Initially, it was determined that Davey had attending skills that allowed him to participate constructively in an activity for approximately four minutes after which time he became restless or disruptive. Therefore, initial periods of activity and instruction were set for approximately this duration with short breaks in between work tasks. This time period was gradually increased to 20 minutes, by gradually expanding the task requirement while maintaining a high interest and success rate. This procedure eliminated the frustration and continuous punishment that is often experienced by children who are expected to attend longer than they are able to perform on a task that is much too long and demanding.

The Utilization of a Response Cost-Techniques for Hitting and Grabbing During the Free Play Period

This technique consisted of the daily presentation of a card of bright animal stickers to Davey prior to the free play period. Each time Davey hit a child or grabbed a toy, a sticker was removed. Davey was allowed to keep the remaining stickers at the end of the period. A variety of other techniques had been used to control hitting and grabbing in some of Davey's other peers in the classroom, however, this particular procedure seemed to be most effective with Davey. He liked to take the stickers home at night and enjoyed playing with them; hence, they served as a good reinforcer for good behavior and a good response cost for inappropriate behavior.

Specific Instruction and Training in Skill Areas in Which Davey was Weak or Deficient

Rather than simply wait for important development skills to emerge as a result of general preschool classroom activity, specific training activities were devised to systematically build such skills. These included specific instruction in playing and manipulating play materials, speech and language skills, fine and gross motor skills, and several pre-academic skills. The gradual development of such skills expanded Davey's repertoire of behavior which he could draw upon in playing with other children. As he gained such skills, Davey began to exhibit them in the classroom as he played with other children.

The Gradual Shift from 1-1 Instruction to
Small and Finally Large Group Arrangements
for Davey's Instructional Programs

All of Davey's initial instructional programs were presented under a 1-1 basis in a non-distracting part of the preschool classroom. As his attending skills were developed and his performance improved, he was moved into small group activities and eventually into large group instructional sessions. As the group structure was changed, Davey was reinforced for taking turns, for working more independently, and for contributing to the group activities.

The Utilization of Relaxation Exercises on a Daily Basis

The relaxation exercises were prescribed by the occupational therapist who worked with the special classroom program to prevent overstimulation and to quiet Davey after high activity periods. Davey was positioned in nonactive sitting and lying postures and put through movement activities. This resulted in a decrease in body tension and an increase in Davey's overall calmness during the exercise period.

As evidenced by the foregoing discussion, the major focus of Davey's treatment program was not directly upon his hyperactive behavior. Instead, it was focused upon the development of behaviors that he needed to perform more successfully in his preschool environment. This was carried out by the individually prescribed training programs for Davey within the total context of a supportive physical, social, and instructional environment. That environment was intentionally structured to minimize the probability that Davey would engage in hyperactive behaviors.

Conclusion

The frequency of occurrences or episodes of hyperactivity decreased significantly in Davey's second preschool classroom environment. Data was recorded on the same behaviors that had been previously observed in the first classroom at the time of his referral. This data was recorded for the first several months of his placement in the second classroom. Davey's roaming behavior did not occur at all in the special classroom. His activities were structured in such a manner that he increasingly became more actively engaged in interactions with peers, teaching staff, and materials in a way that was appropriate to his current functioning level. Previous problems of non-attending and non-compliance to teacher directions were eliminated by systematic training and reinforcement. Similar results were observed in relation to his verbal interruptions. Activities and training programs were designed specifically for Davey and presented at a level which allowed for his successful participation. Only four inappropriate verbal interruptions were recorded during the first month Davey was enrolled in the special program. Davey's mean time for engaging in play and instructional sessions remained at three to four minutes initially. However, this ceased to be a direct problem, since instruction was adapted to his attentional skill level and was scheduled to run for exactly that duration for each task given. The duration of instructional activities was successfully increased to 20 minutes. Davey's hitting and grabbing of play materials from peers continued to appear for a longer period of time and seemed to be related to his lack of social skill in procuring desired toys. The response-cost system eliminated this behavior by the onset of the third month.

A probable explanation for this rather abrupt decrease in hyperactivity is that the total environment was structured in such a way that Davey, as well as the other children had neither the opportunity nor the need to behave in a hyperactive manner. In essence, Davey's behavioral repertoire and the environment were appropriately matched, so that the interaction between Davey and his environment produced positive-growth-producing behavior. This is the basis for the ecological approach to an educational intervention for young handicapped or developmentally delayed children.

After 18 months in the early childhood special education setting, Davey's overall developmental level and behavior suggested that he could make a successful adjustment to a public school setting, provided he receive supportive services from special education.

In summary, an ecological perspective of hyperactivity in preschool handicapped children is based upon several important assumptions as reflected in the description and discussion of Davey's case study. They are as follows:

(1) Behavior and environment are functional components of an interactive system.

(2) Behavior may be viewed as hyperactive, not because of its nature or form, but because there is an inadequate match between an

individual's behavior and instructional needs and his/her educational environment.

(3) Behaviors labeled as hyperactive may be managed by therapeutic strategies that focus upon an individual's behavior within a total ecological system, rather than solely upon the hyperactive behavior itself.

(4) Behaviors labeled hyperactive within a classroom setting are often related to and managed by an individual's interaction with the physical, social, and instructional components of an ecological system.

CASE STUDY #16. TEACHER CONSULTATION AS AN INTERVENTION WITH A HYPERACTIVE SECOND-GRADE BOY

Stephen DeMers and Joy P. Burke

Teacher consultation has long been recognized as an important function in the role of the school psychologist (Bardon, 1963; Gray, 1963; Losen, 1964; Newman, 1967). Also, the school psychologist-teacher (or counselor-teacher, social worker-teacher, etc.) relationship is often the vehicle for the implementation of school interventions with hyperactive children (Fine, 1977; Renshaw, 1974; Ross and Ross, 1976; Valett, 1974). Therefore, it seems appropriate to focus on teacher consultation as a specific intervention that is helpful in working with hyperactive children in school.

Although much has been written, especially recently, on the application of consultation theory to the school environment in general (e.g., Dinkmeyer and Carlson, 1975; Meyers et al., 1977; Parker, 1975), there have been few empirical studies of the effectiveness of consultation and few specific applications of consultation techniques to children's problem behaviors, such as hyperactivity. Several authors have addressed the consultative aspects of implementing behavior-management programs in schools (e.g., Abidin, 1972; Grieger, 1972), and these indirectly relate to the treatment of hyperactivity and other behavioral problems of children. The few empirical studies in the literature (Kaplan and Sprunger, 1967; Meyers et al., 1975; Tyler and Fine, 1974) have demonstrated teacher-consultation strategies to be effective in changing the teachers' understanding of children's behavior problems in a positive direction.

The writings of Gerald Caplan (1963, 1964, 1970), the uncontested "father" of mental health consultation, continue to be the best source of guidance in this area. Caplan (1963) defined consultation as:

A process of interaction between two professional persons—the consultant, who is a specialist, and the consultee, who invokes his help in regard to a current work problem with which the latter is having some difficulty and which he has decided is within the former's area of specialized competence. (p. 470)

A distinctive feature of consultation, however, is the fact that the consultant does not assume responsibility for the client but, instead offers assistance or suggests plans of action to the consultee, who maintains responsibility for the client and who also reserves the right to accept or reject the consultant's suggestions. In the present case, we are interested in focusing on how a process of interaction between a school psychologist, who is the consultant, and a teacher, who is the consultee, can help to reduce the hyperactive behaviors of a student who is the consultee's client.

Caplan (1963, 1970) discusses four basic types of mental health consultation, however, both Caplan (1970) and others (Fine and Tyler, 1971) see one of the four types of consultation as the most relevant to work in schools. This type of consultation is called consultee-centered case consultation and refers to a type of consultation where a consultee's difficulty in handling a particular client seems related, at least in part, to the consultee himself. Caplan (1963) and Fine and Tyler (1971) discuss the following four major categories of difficulty which might interfere with a teacher's ability to resolve a particular child's problem behavior.

(1) *Lack of understanding.* This is the category of consultee difficulty where the teacher "may have drawn erroneous conclusions or may simply lack the psychological skill to draw any conclusions regarding a child's behavior that he finds unusual or disturbing" (Fine and Tyler, 1971, p. 440).

(2) *Lack of skill or information.* In this situation, the teacher's lack of information about how to deal with a specific behavior is the major difficulty.

(3) *Lack of objectivity.* This is where a teacher's personal needs, attitudes, or misconceptions have resulted in some stereotyped view of the child's problem behavior and a consequent inability to deal objectively

with the situation. Caplan (1963) has emphasized this category and used the term "theme-interference" to refer to the consultee's inability to deal with the client's behavior because of his or her own personal "themes."

(4) *Lack of confidnce or self-esteem*. This last category of consultee difficulty refers to the situation in which a consultee just needs some support and/or encouragement from an outside professional to resolve his situation satisfactorily.

In the case of a hyperactive child, it is not difficult to perceive numerous situations in which a teacher (or parent) might have difficulty dealing effectively with a child's restless, inattentive, and distractible behavior because of one or more of these four categories of consultee behaviors. For example, the following are possible sources of teacher inability to deal with a hyperactive child and require teacher consultation to effect change: (a) lack of understanding of the nature or treatment of hyperactivity; (b) a lack of skill in designing an intervention strategy (e.g., behavior modification, prescriptive teaching, perceptual motor training, etc.); (c) lack of objectivity about the uncontrollable nature of most hyperactive behaviors; and/or (d) lack of self-confidence or self-esteem of the teacher who is working with a severely hyperactive child.

Consultee-centered case consultation is conducted by engaging the teacher in a consultation relationship where, although the apparent focus is on the child's problem behavior, the consultant also attempts to effect changes in the teacher (Meyers et al., 1977). First, while discussing the child's problem behavior, the consultant tries to determine which of the four categories of consultee difficulties may be operating. Then, depending on the type of difficulty, the consultant recommends a plan of action and/or offers observations of the problem, which are designed as much to address the teachers lack of understanding or skill, as to specifically deal with the child's problem behavior.

Obviously, this close relationship between the teacher (consultee) and the pyschologist (consultant) requires much time and trust in order to be effective, as well as much skill on the part of the consultant. Description of the specific skills necessary to effectively consult with teachers is beyond the scope of this article, but the reader is referred to the works of Caplan (1963, 1964, 1970), Lippitt (1967), and Rogers (1959).

Teacher consultation often may be just one of a variety of interventions used in any one case of hyperactivity. As Fine and Tyler (1971) point out:

This approach to consultation does not preclude the possibility that the child may be experiencing a "real" problem; it simply emphasizes how a better classroom adjustment might be affected for the child through a change in teacher understanding and behavior. (p. 439)

The following case study presents an example of how teacher consultation aided in the proper intervention with a hyperactive child.

Current Problem

Cliff is a nice-looking, somewhat slightly built, seven-year-old boy who is having considerable difficulty controlling his behavior in the school environment. Cliff is described by his second-grade teacher as being "restless, fidgety, constantly in motion, inattentive in class, and disruptive to the other students." In addition, Cliff frequently "fails to complete his assignments and can be aggressive with other students at times." Academically, Cliff has most difficulty with reading, writing, and language arts, in general; while he seems strong in hands-on, construction-type activities, and verbal expression. Because of his impulsive and, at times, explosive behavior, Cliff has been suspended from school several times. Numerous parent conferences have been held and finally, Cliff was referred for both a medical and psychological evaluation in the hope that some medication would be prescribed that could control his behavior.

Background Information

Cliff is the second oldest of four sons from an intact, middle-class family. Cliff's father is an engineer and his mother is a former elementary school teacher. Cliff's parents are quite concerned about his school difficulties, especially since his older brother is a fine student and the two younger boys are already showing academic and social skills to rival Cliff's. Cliff's mother stated in fact that she is embarrassed that Cliff is not meeting the family's expectations for school achievement.

After the second parent conference, Cliff's parents and teacher concluded that he should be seen by the local pediatrician and probably medicated to control his hyperactive behaviors. A routine psychological evaluation was requested to confirm the diagnosis of hyperactivity.

Results of the psychological evaluation revealed the following. On the *Behavior Problem Checklist* completed by both the parents and the teacher, Cliff was rated highest on the following dimensions: restlessness; disruptiveness; short-attentiveness; hyperactivity; and distractibility. Observation of Cliff in the classroom and on the playground by the school psychologist suggested that indeed he did have problems of inattention, distractibility, poor impulse control, and other features of the hyperactive syndrome. On the WISC-R, Cliff earned a Full Scale of 99 with Verbal IQ equal to 106 and Performance IQ equal to 91, indicating average intellectual ability. However, the discrepancy between verbal and performance IQ, as well as the relative strengths in vocabulary and verbal abstract reasoning did not seem to adequately explain Cliff's difficulties in reading and language arts.

In view of his relative weaknesses in visual completion and copying tasks, one possible conclusion was that Cliff's problems with reading and writing might be based on a perceptual-motor rather than language-arts deficit. The results of the Bender-Gestalt confirmed an approximate two-year delay in Cliff's perceptual-motor maturation. Additional psychoneurological screening tasks suggested difficulty with eye-hand coordination and visual tracking. Personality assessment of Cliff suggested high anxiety and insecurity, as well as strong feelings of inadequacy and some hostility.

Results of the pediatric evaluation were essentially negative with no evidence of either minimal brain dysfunction or other neurological impairments. However, in consultation with the psychologist, it was recommended that Cliff be seen by a developmental opthamologist who, after extensive assessment, determined that Cliff had a relatively severe eye-tracking problem. It was suggested that this visual tracking problem could easily account for Cliff's difficulty with reading, writing, and other skills requiring such eye-hand coordination, and that the continual frustration might account for Cliff's short attention span, distractibility, incomplete assignments, and other "hyperactive behavior." A remediation program at a private clinic was begun immediately and both the pediatrician and opthamologist sent reports to the parents and the school describing Cliff's difficulties and the treatment program to be implemented.

The parents readily accepted this explanation of Cliff's academic difficulties, however, the school, and especially Cliff's teacher, responded to the physicians' reports as "double talk," since they all knew Cliff was one of those "hyperactive kids who needs medication." After Cliff had been going to the private clinic weekly for about two months, he began to show improved eye-tracking skill and began reading at home and becoming less troublesome. In school, however, Cliff continued to have the same difficulties as before, which the school staff and Cliff's teacher regarded as evidence that Cliff still needed to be medicated. In effect, it appeared that a pattern of shared expectations had developed between Cliff and the school, such that even when his original difficulty was remediated, the old behaviors were still maintained by the environment.

The school psychologist in this situation came to the conclusion that what had began as a case of a boy with perceptual difficulties who evidenced some hyperactive behaviors in response to his academic and social failures, ultimately became a problem of what Caplan (1963) referred to as "theme interference." As noted earlier, theme interference refers to the situation in which a primary caretaker cannot appropriately deal with a client's problem behavior because of some misconception of the situation or misinformation about the nature of the problem behavior. In this case, Cliff's teacher was apparently unwittingly maintaining Cliff's hyperactive behaviors because of the faulty belief that these behaviors were to be expected until Cliff was medicated.

Intervention

According to Caplan's (1963) theory of mental health consultation, theme interference is removed through a process of consultee-centered, case consultation in which the goal of the consulting relationship is as much to change the behavior of the primary caretaker (or consultee) as to change the client's behavior. This is accomplished by discovering which of four common sources of consultee difficulty is in operation. In this case, Cliff's teacher seemed to be evidencing the type of theme interference known as "lack of understanding of the psychological factors" inherent in the problem behavior and a lack of objectivity in Cliff's problem behavior. That is, Cliff's teacher seemed to have a lack of understanding of the multifaceted nature of hyperactive behaviors and instead held a stereotypic view that all hyperactive children must be medicated. The intervention required, therefore, that the school psychologist or other appropriate consultant offer a consultative relationship to this teacher, whereby in the process of discussing and helping to change the client's behavior, the goal is also to reduce or eliminate the teacher's lack of understanding of the nature and treatment of hyperactive behavior in children, in general, and Cliff, in particular.

The specific intervention in this case consisted of a combination of a general in-service education program for all school staff on the topic of hyperactivity in which the goal was to provide factual information about the problem, in general; and, secondly, a behavior-management program for Cliff's teacher to deal with Cliff in the classroom, with the goal of breaking the pattern of shared expectations of hyperactive behavior. The in-service education program was suggested because it appeared that Cliff's teacher was not alone in the belief that all hyperactive children need medication. Therefore, all the teachers needed to be involved to lessen the likelihood of group pressure undermining the consultant's work with Cliff's teacher and also, as an efficient mechanism for possibly preventing similar situations in the future.

The in-service program consisted of a 2½-hour presentation offered for teachers during one afternoon at the school, and included presentations by a school psychologist, pediatrician, and dietician. Each presented a brief description of how specific deficits or deficiencies in their particular area of expertise could contribute to hyperactive behaviors in children. Each also discussed the treatment or intervention programs available. The focus of the program was on the multi-dimensional nature of hyperactivity and its remediation. Some reading material about hyperactivity was excerpted from major texts on the topic and provided to participants. A question-and-answer period, as well as an evaluation form administered at the conclusion of the session, provided clear evidence of a broadening of participant viewpoints about hyperactivity.

A few days before the workshop, Cliff's teacher and the school psychologist developed a rather typical behavior modification program, following the teachers' complaint that "nothing was being done for Cliff since he was refused medication." In consultation with the school psychologist, the teacher selected out-of-seat behavior, incomplete assignments, and verbal outbursts as target behaviors. Reinforcement for improved performance included charting with "stars," teacher praise, and participation in special activities chosen from a reinforcement menu.

Within five school days, Cliff's target behaviors had been eliminated as sources of concern for his teacher. He also began reading, attending, and generally achieving and not disrupting the class. The behavior management program was discontinued to determine if the program was the cause of Cliff's behavior change. The problem behaviors did not return after the program ended, suggesting that with remediation of his eye-tracking difficulties, Cliff was capable of adjusting and achieving in school, once he and his teacher were motivated to change their pattern of interaction.

Cliff's teacher subsequently reported her pleasure with the change in Cliff and her recognition that medication was not always necessary to deal with hyperactive behaviors in children.

Conclusion

This case study describes a situation in which teacher consultation was necessary to effectively reduce the hyperactive behaviors of a second-grade boy. However, teacher-consultation techniques are applicable whenever one suspects that a parent, teacher, administrator, etc., may hold a stereotypic or faulty view of hyperactivity, with theme interference operating to prevent successful resolution of the child's problem behavior. The specifics of the teacher-consultation approach will vary depending on the nature of the problem and the setting in which the consultation is to take place. Several new books have recently become available to aid those unfamiliar with the various techniques of teacher consultation, including Meyers et al. (1977), Dinkmeyer and Carlson, (1975), and Parker (1974).

References

ABIDIN, R. A psychosocial look at consultation and behavior modification. *Psychol. in the Schools.* 1972, 9(4):358-364.

BARDON, J. I. Mental health education: A framework for psychological services in the schools. *J. School Psychol.* 1963, 1:20-27.

CAPLAN, G. Types of mental health consultation. *Amer. J. Orthopsychiat.* 1963, 33: 470-481.

CAPLAN, G. *Principles of Preventive Psychiatry.* New York: Basic Books, 1970.

CAPLAN, G. *The Theory and Practice of Mental Health Consultation.* New York: Basic Books, 1970.

DINKMEYER, D. and CARLSON, J. (eds.). *Consultation: A Book of Readings.* New York: John Wiley, 1975.

FINE, M. (ed.). *Principles and Techniques of Intervention with Hyperactive Children.* Springfield, Ill.: Charles C Thomas, 1977.

FINE, M. and TYLER, M. Concerns and directions in teacher consultation. *J. School Psychol.* 1971, 9:436-444.

GRAY, S. W. *The Psychologist in the Schools.* New York: Holt, Rinehart, & Winston, 1963.

GRIEGER, R. Teacher attitudes as a variable in behavior modification consultation. *J. School Psychol.* 1972, 10:279-287.

KAPLAN, M. and SPRUNGER, B. Psychological evaluations and teacher perception of students. *J. School Psychol.* 1967, 5:287-291.

LIPPITT, G. L. The consultative process. *The School Psychol.* 1967, 21:72-74.

LOSEN, S. M. The school psychologist-psychotherapist or consultant. *Psychol. in the Schools* 1964, 1:13-17.

MEYERS, J., FREIDMAN, M., and GAUGHAN, E., JR. The effects of consultee-centered consultation on teacher behavior. *Psychol. in the Schools.* 1975, 12(3):288-295.

MEYERS, J., MARTIN, R., and HYMAN, I. (eds.). *School Consultation: Readings About Preventive Techniques for Pupil Personnel Workers.* Springfield, Ill.: Charles C Thomas, 1977.

NEWMAN, R. G. *Psychological Consultation in the Schools.* New York: Basic Books, 1967.

PARKER, C. (ed.). *Psychological Consultation: Helping Teachers Meet Special Needs.* Reston, Va.: Council for Exceptional Children, 1975.

RENSHAW, S. *The Hyperactive Child.* Chicago: Nelson-Hall, 1974.

ROGERS, C. R. Significant learning: In therapy and education. *Educa. Leadership* 1959, 16:232-242.

Ross, D. M. and Ross, S. A. *Hyperactivity: Research, Theory and Action.* New York: John Wiley, 1976.

TYLER, M. and FINE, M. J. The effects of limited and intensive school psychologist-teacher consultation. *J. School Psychol.* 1974, 12:8-16.

VALETT, R. E. *The Psychoeducational Treatment of Hyperactive Children.* Belmont, Ca.: Fearon Publishers, 1974.

CHAPTER 7

Psychotherapeutic
Intervention

The definition, goals, and procedures of psychotherapy are difficult to define in ways that would satisfy the practitioners and theoreticians of psychotherapy. In the traditional image, we find a therapist listening empathically, occasionally offering interpretations, and otherwise involved in building a supportive relationship with the client. The contemporary variations of therapy include differing theoretical orientations and procedures; group and family, as well as individual treatment; a range of active to passive involvement by therapist and client; and variations of time in therapy.

Psychotherapy in isolation from other interventions has not been a popular modality of treatment for hyperactive children. Wender (1973) makes some very strong statements, supported by others (Cantwell, 1975; and Stewart and Olds, 1973) that "There are no data whatsoever supporting the usefulness of psychotherapy in the basic treatment of hyperactive children" (p. 102).

There is recognition, however, that the patterns of hyperactivity can affect the child's personal and social adjustment and bring stress to family and school settings. Psychotherapy is seen more positively as a vehicle for helping involved persons cope with the hyperactive child in their charge, and also to directly assist the hyperactive child in coping with such

173

secondary symptoms as low self-esteem, depression, anger, and poor peer relationships.

The negative view espoused by Wender (1973) seems based on his belief that the cause of hyperactivity was mainly constitutional, rather than emotional. There are positions stated in the literature arguing that some patterns of hyperactivity may well be emotionally based, either as a reaction to stress, or as a means of the child's coping with his environment (Palmer, 1970; Averswald, 1969; Marwitt and Stenner, 1972; and Friedland and Shilkret, 1973). In these instances, psychotherapy would seem justified as a main or adjunct treatment.

Another way that psychotherapy, broadly interpreted, enters the treatment situation is through the attitudes of the persons involved. By acting out an empathic and caring relationship with the hyperactive child, the "help" person, be he teacher, clinician or parent, is conveying some very important messages to the child. The child is more likely to develop positive feelings about himself under these conditions and develop the internal strengths to cope with day-to-day stress.

Structural family theory (Minuchin, 1974) views symptoms in the context of the family system. The case study presented on family therapy intervention illustrates how hyperactivity, as a symptom pattern, can be connected to family dysfunction. With mental health professionals and educators "rediscovering" the family, this is a particularly appropriate and stimulating study to be included. The second case study demonstrates a therapeutic orientation to an eclectic approach. This includes involving the parents in a counseling program, as well as the teachers and other personnel responding sensitively to the child's feelings and emotional needs.

Both case studies offer the reader a picture of the diversity of theories and procedures related to therapeutic intervention.

References

AVERSWALD, E. H. Cognitive development and psychopathology in the urban environment. In Graubard, P. S. (ed.), *Children Against the Schools*. Chicago: Follett, 1969.

CANTWELL, D. P. *The Hyperactive Child: Diagnosis, Management, Current Research*. New York: Spectrum Publications, 1975.

FRIEDLAND, S. J. and SHILKRET, R. B. Alternative explanations of learning disabilities: Defensive hyperactivity. *Except. Child.* 1973, 40:213-215.

MARWITT, S. J. and STENNER, A. J. Hyperkinesis: Delineation of two patterns. *Except. Child.* 1972, 38:401-406.

MINUCHIN, S. *Families and Family Therapy*. Cambridge, Mass.: Harvard University Press, 1974.

PALMER, J. O. *The Psychological Assessment of Children.* New York: Wiley, 1970.
STEWART, M. A. and OLDS, S. W. *Raising a Hyperactive Child.* New York: Harper & Row, 1973.
WENDER, P. H. *The Hyperactive Child: A Handbook for Parents.* New York: Crown Publishers, 1973.

CASE STUDY #17. A THERAPEUTIC, MULTI-FACETED INTERVENTION PROGRAM WITH A PRESCHOOL HYPERACTIVE BOY

Linda H. Jackson

The Pre-School Day Treatment Center of The Menninger Foundation is a therapeutic nursery and kindergarten for children two and one-half to six years of age, with largely medical and psychodynamic orientation. Drawing from psychoanalytic and ego psychological models, an attempt is made to integrate other approaches, including behavior modification, and child development. Classes are small, with approximately 10 children in the morning preschool and another ten in afternoon kindergarten. Two or three staff teachers, and one or more student teachers provide high staff/pupil ratio, allowing for individual and small group work on feelings, socialization, play, and academic work. Each child's treatment is individually planned by the staff and coordinated by a child psychiatrist team leader.

Although our preschool was set up for children with emotional problems of varying degrees, we frequently have children with mild to moderate learning disabilities and/or neurological or other handicaps. Hyperactivity is a frequent symptom among our referrals; some of the hyperactive children have appeared to be primarily emotionally disturbed, and some have appeared to be primarily brain damaged, with emotional disturbance secondary to the problems of coping with abnormal brain function. In order to meet the needs of the disturbed, deprived, or multiply handicapped children, the staff has attempted to develop a flexible, multidisciplinary program; emphasizing the medical-neurological, social, behavioral, educational, family, emotional, and recreational aspects of the child's development. Moreover, since the child spends the major part of his day interacting with his family, the parents are considered to be an integral part of the treatment team. Parents meet regularly with staff to plan treatment goals and to work together to effect changes.

Each child is evaluated during the first few weeks, and an individualized treatment program is worked out for him. There is no "typical" case. The case of R. is given as an example of how we treated one hyperactive child with a multidisciplinary approach.

Current Problem

R. is a three-year-old boy referred for intervention in a therapeutic preschool setting by his pediatrician, because of his slow motor development and hyperactivity. R.'s mother is very concerned about R.'s hyperactivity, clumsiness, short attention span, and restlessness; but she feels that his cognitive development is appropriate.

R. is generally healthy physically, except for strabismus and refractive errors. He has staring spells, drools slightly, and has unintelligible speech. He is a rather plain looking boy, of average size, who is extremely restless and clumsy. He falls frequently when playing, but does not seem concerned about his falls, even when injured. In fact, he does not show much emotion generally. He goes from one activity to another quickly, with a short attention span (a few seconds) for any one toy or activity. The interviewing room is strewn with toys in no time. He does not have hand dominance, and has poor small muscle coordination as well as large motor difficulties.

He appears to have a good, but "frayed" relationship with his mother and other members of the family, although his short attention span makes mutual activities difficult. His speech is unintelligible except to his mother, although he clearly understands what others say to him and uses sentences of adequate length of his age. His mother reports that he responds to affection but not to discipline. R. sleeps only five hours a night—at most— and does not take naps. He is toilet trained, feeds himself, and can unbutton and button his clothes. He does not yet attempt to play with other children.

Background Information

There were no known abnormalities with the pregnancy or delivery of the child. As an infant, R. was restless, slept very little, and had frequent staring spells. Developmental milestones were on the slow side of average, with walking occurring at 14 months. R.'s gait, balance, and muscle control have continued to be poorly coordinated.

R.'s family has had various problems for the last few years, although the family appears more stable now than previously. The parents, both well educated, were divorced two years ago. R. and his mother now live with the extended family. There is minimal contact between R. and his father.

Prior to his referral, R. had had a brief, unsuccessful trial of Dextro-amphetamine, and there were consultations with a neurologist, ophthal-mologist, and speech pathologist. Electroencephalogram and echogram were normal. The ophthalmologist plans eyeglasses and a patching program to improve central fixation and acuity, but has difficulty planning an appro-priate refraction because of R.'s inability to cooperate during testing. The speech pathologist did not find organic components in his speech disturb-ance, and recommended therapeutic nursery school rather than speech therapy at this time. Hearing could not be tested, as R. was too hyperactive to cooperate, even on a second visit, when a sedative was given.

Diagnostic impression at the time of admission was 309.9. Nonpsychotic Organic Brain Syndrome was characterized by hyperactivity, short attention span, and poor fine and gross motor development, as well as Esotropia of the left eye.

Intervention

The following treatment plan was subsequently developed: R. was to begin attending the therapeutic preschool for half-day periods, in order to participate in a therapeutic group experience and to have further assess-ments of his strength and limitations. This evaluation would include further educational assessment, learning disabilities screening, assessment of anxiety, and further assessment of hearing and vision when the child could better cooperate. His mother would participate in weekly individual parent guid-ance sessions, which at times included the whole family. (Note: In two-parent families, both parents are involved in parent guidance.) In addition, the mother would be encouraged to join a parents' group. She would be encouraged to observe R. in the school setting, and, having many assets herself, would be coached in helping R. to understand and master his assets and liabilities, and assisting him in remediation programs. A diagnostic family interview would be held to help determine how the extended family might be involved in the treatment. Consideration would be given to use of medication. R. would have remediation activities in use of large and small muscles and coordination. In addition, use would be made of play and verbalization to help R. understand his feelings.

R. began attending nursery school in the middle of the semester. He had some separation problems at first; he refused to accept much adult help, and was very hyperactive. After he had been coming long enough for the staff to determine his behavior baseline, R. was started on medication (Methyl-phenidate). Eventually, after many trials and errors, a dosage was found which enabled him to slow down slightly, at least enough to sleep for eight hours at night, without untoward effects.

Since R. was frequently testing limits and threatening temper tantrums, his teachers used a firm approach; insisting that he follow limits and try more self-help tasks, encouraging him to verbalize feelings instead of kicking, and using positive reinforcement liberally. The family was encouraged to use similar methods as well as to look for things to praise. With gradual increases of expectations for longer periods of concentration (e.g. for sitting and listening at story time), R.'s attention span also gradually increased.

For large motor development, R. was encouraged to slow down and focus on where he wanted to go before he took off, and was given individual work with large movements. Reminding him to slow down and watch where he was aiming, helped R. to decrease the incidence of falls. Both teachers and family worked on this with R. His mother was asked to have him wear tennis shoes instead of cowboy boots, to help some with balance. R. was also given individual instruction in small muscle activity; such as cutting with scissors, playing with clay, and Frostig material.

Using candy as a reinforcer, the teachers taught R. how to point out the directions of the "E's" on the vision chart, so that he could be retested and fitted with glasses. Combined efforts of both his home and school were necessary to get R. to wear his glasses. However, as R. wore the glasses more and had better use of his eyes, his movements developed more purpose, and he appreciated staff efforts to find him the best place to view books and slides.

After a few months at school, the teachers noted that R.'s self-esteem was suffering, due to his comparing himself to others. A program was devised whereby R. was given activities in which he could be successful, i.e., if the class was to be doing an activity that was too difficult for R. to do without great frustration, he would be separated from the others and given an individual task within his capability. As with other techniques, this plan was shared with R.'s mother, who attempted to implement it at home as well. Both teachers and mother praised R. for his work. R. blossomed under this program, became more trusting and affectionate, and developed some self-confidence, so that his frustration tolerance increased and he gradually became able to try harder tasks.

Meanwhile, in the weekly parent guidance sessions, R.'s mother was helped to talk about her natural frustrations in working with such a difficult child, the disappointments in having a child with handicapps, the emotional acceptance of R.'s problems and strengths, and the guilt feelings involved in allowing the child to separate from her and develop autonomy.

Also in the parent guidance sessions, feedback was shared so that any new or promising techniques begun either at home or in school could be tried at both places. It was stressed that approaches be as consistent as possible, responses noted, and stressful events (death of a pet, leaving of a staff member, trips, etc.) be known about and dealt with both at home and school.

In family sessions, work focused on the inevitable frustrations all family members experienced in having to live with R., attempts to plan practical ways of dealing with him more effectively at home, and allowing family members to deal with their own feelings without taking them out on R. His mother was encouraged to have a baby-sitter from time to time, so as to have some relaxation without unduly burdening herself or other family members. R.'s mother voluntarily participated in a parents' group, where she and the other parents could give each other mutual support. She was instrumental in developing educational programs on topics, such as learning disabilities, for the group. After six months in the preschool, R. was referred to a motor-development program at another institution, which he attended while continuing in his program at the preschool.

R.'s speech continued to be characterized by articulation errors. Repeated hearing testing showed normal peripheral hearing. With knowledge of the central auditory discrimination problem, staff members could work in the classroom and with the family to provide instructions for R. in a simple, slowly stated manner, with a minimum of distracting background noise (e.g. take him aside and turn off the TV). As he approached four years of age, R. began to become interested in playing with other children. At first, he would sit by himself and scream that he had no one to play with; but the teachers encouraged him to ask the other children to play. He clumsily began playing with others and developed a friendship with another little boy, whom he followed and imitated.

During this first year, R.'s attention span increased, as did his ability to express emotions. His clumsiness and negativism decreased. His speech improved as his anxiety lessened.

After one year medication was stopped for a "drug holiday."[1] No gains were lost and there were no regressions while off medication. So, medication was discontinued.

After 15 months in the preschool, R. was transferred to the therapeutic

---

[1] "Drug holiday" refers to a planned time off from long-term medication such as amphetamines to allow for normal growth to take place, as these medications sometimes interfere with physical growth.

kindergarten. Although he had made good progress during the past year, this was a difficult year for R., due to added stress in his home (a long serious illness of a family member), and to his increasing awareness of his limitations. His former best friend in the group had advanced faster than he had, leaving R. lonley. However, by this time R.'s attention span had increased enough so that he could apply himself well to academic work and take pride in his cognitive accomplishments and the papers which he could take home.

R. found a new friend and went through a stage of idealizing, imitating, and serving his friend. At the same time, he went through a phase of playing "disaster," (i.e., of pretending to be a victim of all kinds of "accidents" and having to be rescued by police, firemen, superheroes, etc.). The therapy team attempted to reinforce his independent and appropriate skills so that he would not have to be so dependent and clinging in his peer relations. For example, they told him that they liked him when he behaved like himself better than when he copied his friend. The teachers also tried to make him understand that he did not have to be either badly hurt or super-skilled to be liked and cared for. Later in the year, R. gave up his clinging, idealizing relationship to the other boy and behaved more appropriately but, being unable to keep up with most of the other children, was again a loner. He became sulky and negativistic at school. His sulking was ignored, and expectations were maintained at his level. Teachers tried to encourage him to talk about his loneliness and discouragement, rather than acting it out by negative behavior.

Parallel to these concerns of R. during these months, his mother was working in her parent guidance process and parent group on feelings of discouragement, lack of community support, and worries about R.'s future. As she coped with these difficulties, she was instrumental in working with community groups for improvement of learning resources for disabled children.

In liaison with the public schools, a plan was worked out whereby R. would attend regular kindergarten, (since there was no special education available in his district) with some help from a learning disabilities resource teacher, mornings and would return to the therapeutic kindergarten afternoons during the first several weeks of school, until he was well adjusted. This plan was accomplished, with the teachers from the two schools maintaining close contact.

R. adjusted very well to his public school classroom. In the afternoon therapeutic kindergarten program, he became a kind of a teacher's helper and a leader in the group. As soon as it was apparent that R. had adjusted to the public school classroom, his termination date was scheduled, allowing ample time to prepare both R. and his long-time peers for the separation. Ambivalence and anxiety over losing the support of the program caused much last-minute limit testing and some tantrum behavior. Staff empathy with his fears of failure, as well as support for his achievements, seemed to ease much of his distress and he was amply settled down by his last week. On his final day, he could talk about being ready to go to the "grown-up" school and could accept praise for the great progress he had made.

Plans were for him to continue in the public school classroom, with learning resources and speech therapy available. The family was to continue some work with the counselor.

Conclusion

R., a severely hyperactive child with some brain damage, responded to a multifaceted program that included therapeutic group interactions, individualized training in coordination, parent guidance, medication and positive reinforcement combined with ophthalmologic care. An adjunctive motor development program in another setting was also included.

Especially helpful in working with this child was the fact that the staff initially cut out as many of the circumstances which would lead to failure as possible; introducing R. to things in which he could succeed, and gradually adding more difficult tasks. This program grew out of both the staff and family empathizing with the great amount of difficulty this child had in relating to his environment and to other people.

References

ACK, M., BEALE, E., and WARE, L. Parent guidance: Psychotherapy of the young child via the parent. *Bull. Menninger Clin.* 1975, 39:436-447.

BRUTTEN, M., RICHARDSON, S. O., and MANGEL, C. *Something's Wrong With My Child.* New York: Harcourt, Brace & Jovanovich, 1973.

CIBA: MBD Compendium, (Series of articles on Minimal Brain Dysfunction from multidisciplinary approach.) Ciba Pharmaceutical Company, Summit, New Jersey, 07901.

ERIKSON, E. *Childhood and Society* (2nd Ed.). New York: Norton, 1963.

FRAIBERG, S. *The Magic Years.* New York: Charles Scribner's, 1959.

GARDNER, R. A. *MBD, the Family Book About Minimal Brain Dysfunction.* New York: Aronson, 1973.

MAHLER, M. On the significance of the normal separation-individuation phase. In *Drives, Affects and Behavior,* Vol. 2. New York: International Universities Press, 1965.

MORROW, T. Flexibility in therapeutic work with parents and children. *Bull. Menninger Clin.* 1974, 38:129-143.

PELLER, L. Libidinal phases, ego development and play. *Psychoanalytic Study of the Child*, 1954, 9:178-196.

SEN, M. and SOLNIT, A. *Problems in Child Behavior and Development*. Philadelphia: Lea & Febiger, 1968.

CASE STUDY #18. STRUCTURAL FAMILY THERAPY WITH THE FAMILY OF A HYPERACTIVE CHILD

Katherine G. Kent

In surveying the literature on hyperactive children and their families, most authorities seem to recognize an emotional component to the disorder. Some authors go so far as to state that symptoms usually associated with hyperactivity may be derived purely from emotional factors. For example, one Canadian study (Ney, 1974) outlines four "types" of hyperactivity, including "behavioral" (conditioned) hyperactivity, which is attributed to parents responding selectively to the child's behavior. Another "type" is "reactive" (chaotic) hyperactivity, a diagnosis which is ascribed to children from home environments in which there is little agreement on discipline, or where there is considerable marital turmoil.

While most authorities do not seem willing to define the syndrome this broadly, but, rather, see hyperactivity as having strong genetic determinants with or without traumatic pregnancy and/or birth, all concede that the child's behavior is stressful and often associated with other psychiatric problems, whether in the child or other family members (Cantwell, 1972; Feighner and Feighner, 1974; Welner et al., 1977). Thus, various authors (Safer and Allen, 1976; Stewart and Olds, 1973) emphasize the need for some type of therapeutic intervention, usually of an educational nature, with the child. Parent counseling, also usually an educational type of procedure, is frequently mentioned as a treatment of choice (Safer and Allen ,1976; Stewart and Olds, 1973).

Numerous authors (Safer and Allen, 1976; Cantwell, 1975) note that symptoms of hyperactivity do not seem refractive to formal individual psychotherapy. It seems surprising that Ross and Ross (1976) in their recent volume, *Hyperactivity,* are the only authorities to date to offer a perspective that views family therapy as a highly effective procedure in cases of hyperactivity. Ross and Ross speak to the effectiveness of the brief therapy procedures developed by Weakland and his associates at the Mental Research Institute in Palo Alto, and describe in detail one case treated with this method. They also make references to Boszormenyi-Nagy, Framo, Ferber, Mendellsohn, and Napier as other family therapists whose methods are productive in the treatment of hyperactivity, but do not elaborate their work.

Perhaps one of the major points to be made in detailing a rationale for family therapy as a choice treatment for hyperactive children and their families, is the benefit in choosing a cybernetic model for the understanding of such problems—as opposed to the linear model, which is most frequently used to understand the difficulties of hyperactive children in the literature, to date. Most family therapists use a cybernetic, or systemic model, and find it difficult to derive a functional understanding of problems by using a deductive, cause-and-effect process. Rather, any problem with behavioral manifestations is seen as merely one way of interacting with other members of a system, in a circularity of interactions that is comprised of inevitable simultaneous events. A specific behavior represents a choice an individual makes, to express his/her stake in the outcome of family decisions.

It is assumed by family therapists, that people constantly effect and are, in turn, affected by each other. Thus they maintain an ecological balance which is sometimes shifting and sometimes, in families under stress, maintained by more rigid patterns of interaction. The clinician tries to observe the symptoms produced by the interaction of various systems—including each individual family member, as well as the interplay of biological and emotional systems. The therapist, having observed the habitual patterns of communication that perpetuate a problem, seeks to intervene in a way that blocks the family from reacting in the typical ways which reinforce troublesome behaviors, thus freeing them to seek more constructive solutions.

There are various "brands" of family therapy deriving from a systemic base, that can be useful in the treatment of hyperactivity. In this article, the plan is to discuss the applications of structural family therapy, the modality developed at the Philadelphia Child Guidance Clinic, under the leadership of Salvadore Minuchin and his colleagues. Experience in using this method with hyperactive children and their families leads us to believe that it is particularly effective in such cases.

Structural family therapy is a method which is, initially, highly focused on the specific problem that brings the family for help. It seeks to alleviate the present problem in such a way that new difficulties do not develop in the identified patient or other family members. The aim of the therapy is to bring about a shift in the unspoken rules, or assumptions which govern the behaviors of family members toward one another, and, specifically, to interrupt the circular dysfunctional sequences which produce symptoms. Sessions generally involve all family members that live in the home and the therapist quickly tries to determine whether members of one sub-system, or generation respect the boundaries or functions of the other subsystems. That is, children interfering with parents' efforts to function together as spouses and parents, and parents interferring in their children's efforts to compete and socialize.

It is important to determine where the power, or influence in decision making lies in the family. This is determined by discovering what sorts of alliances and/or coalitions exist within the family; who sides with whom about what. The therapist elicits this data by asking the family members to interact during the interview concerning those problems which bring them for help. They are asked to give their opinions about the problem, each in turn, and then to openly discuss and seek solutions for their disagreements about both the problem and its solutions. In this way, hidden coalitions emerge and the therapist gains enough information to proceed in planning the course of treatment. When certain alliances in the family have become stereotyped and rigid, when certain people always relate only to certain other people and never to others, then the therapist plans to help people shift alliances and roles in a way that will make them able to handle problems in a more flexible way. Tasks which have a paradoxical element that is designed to counter resistance, may be assigned as "homework," as the therapist seeks to continue influencing the modus operandi of the family outside of the structured hour. Thus, the structure of the family is comprised of the patterns of interaction in the family, and the way the family shifts into various camps in the process of trying to solve a problem. It is assumed by the therapist, that this structure must be shifted in those situations in which it has become rigidified, and therefore produced problems which are maintained by the same circularity of interaction.

Structural family therapy seems to be particularly promising for hyperactive children and their families, partly because the difficulties which bring these families for help tend to be concrete and specific, and, thus, lend themselves quite well to the highly focused nature of this treatment. It has long been established that marriages are often and easily stressed by a child's handicap, and it is our experience with hyperactive children and their families that, in many if not all cases that come for help, the parents repeatedly find themselves at odds in attempting to make decisions concerning expectations for their child. Often, one parent is the firm disciplinarian, while the other one is sympathic and overprotective. Interestingly enough, depending upon stresses on individuals in the family, the parents often shift these positions from time to time.

The important thing, is that the parents have difficulty getting together, often because the stress of the child's difficulties enhances latent conflict in the marriage and brings it to the fore, to be enacted around disagreement regarding the child. We could also say that conflict in the marital dyad reinforces the latent propensity in the child towards hyperactivity. In such cases, structural family therapy easily provides a format in which the parents are required, in the presence of the child, to work together towards solutions. It is particularly valuable to have them work on solutions in the present and to attempt to help the child deal with his behavior and the consequences of it. When this happens, the therapist has an optimal opportunity to observe the patterns in the family which lead to reinforcement of both the child's problem and the simultaneous difficulties of other family members. It is one thing to have parents report their interaction in the absence of the child, and another to observe it, and proceed to influence it immediately. It is largely on this basis that we understand the effectiveness that we have had with this method.

Current Problem

Nathan B., age 5 years, 10 months, was referred for diagnostic evaluation by his pediatrician, who in the referral letter described him as "the only truly hyperactive child I have ever seen in my practice." His parents reported that Nathan was constantly active and unable to concentrate on any activity long enough to be productive. He was aggressive and frequently destructive with his toys and other property. Other children in the neighborhood were often forbidden to play with him. Nathan's parents did not allow him to play in the yard without supervision, because he quickly disappeared and, on several occasions, could not be found for hours. His impulsivity led to frequent trips to the emergency room for stitches, and, twice in the past year, he had narrowly missed being hit by a car after darting into the street without looking. Firemen had retrieved him from the roof of the family's home more than once.

Several years ago, the parents stopped taking him to social events and restaurants, because they found it impossible to relax or control him in such situations. A year ago, they had enrolled him in the only pre-school class for developmentally disabled in their town. Almost all of the other children in the class were retarded or had rather severe neurological handicaps. While the teachers noted that Nathan seemed to learn quickly when given individual attention, they expressed frustration and impatience with the task of trying to meet the needs of this one child whose needs seemed to be so different from the others. The school, parents, and pediatrician were interested in the results of our evaluation in order to determine whether Nathan's problems were emotional, neurological or both, and what sort of educational plans should be made for him.

Background Information

Nathan is the only child of a young attorney and his wife, a homemaker. They had tried to conceive for five years prior to the pregnancy, which they recalled as uneventful. Nathan was a full-term infant and delivery was uncomplicated. However, the parents immediately found him to be an intense, demanding child. He slept fitfully at night and seldom during the day. Developmentally, he was precocious; he walked at nine and one-half months, and talked before one year. His parents considered him agile and well coordinated, as exemplified by his ability to climb to the roof of their house. They were convinced that his intelligence was at least normal, but were greatly concerned about his ability to function in kindergarten a few months after he began, due to his distractibility and disruptive behavior.

The pediatrician had tried varying doses of Ritalin, which seemed to help early in the day, only to be followed by an intense period of over-activity late in the afternoon, after the medication had worn off. The parents were concerned because Nathan had lost considerable weight, approximately five pounds in the last year, and had an emaciated look, sunken eyes, and very poor appetite. They had not been informed that the latter symptoms could be a side effect of the Ritalin.

His mother considered herself helpless in controlling Nathan and recounted numerous examples of her fruitless attempts to influence the boy, which usually ended in his doing as he pleased while she shouted and cried. His father was sharply critical of the mother and felt that the problem merely required more patience on her part. He expressed admiration for Nathan's feats of daring and was extremely affectionate with his son, whom he frequently carried in his arms like a small child. He denied much of the signfiicance his wife attributed to the problem, although he also did not attempt to take the child in public. The father stated repeatedly that he had been "just like Nathan" as a child and that more patience would have solved his problem also. He felt sure that the boy would "outgrow it," though he worried about schooling in the meantime.

Intervention

In addition to family sessions, Nathan was seen for an evaluation which included extensive psychological testing and neurological examination. These test result were essentially normal, and he achieved a full-scale IQ of 112. The psychological examiner noted that his intellectual potential was possibly higher, but found it difficult to test him due to his distractibility. His mother was in the room with Nathan during the testing. The parents were asked to take the child off of all medications for the 10-day period of the evaluation and brief treatment.

Nathan and his parents were seen for a total of six one-hour family sessions over a period of 10 days. They had traveled considerable distance to come to the clinic and lived in a motel during this time. The parents were extremely tense in the first session and described their frustration in trying to contain Nathan in a motel room. They felt especially confined in trying to eat meals in the room, since they were sure they could not control him in a restaurant.

After five minutes into the first session, Nathan had begun his exploration of the room and was beginning to climb the bookshelves. In order to determine the structure of this family, and, specifically, the pattern of the interaction in which Nathan's hyperactivity was expressed, the therapist immediately requested that the parents help Nathan to settle down so the interview could proceed. After some expression of surprise and uncertainty, the mother began to ask Nathan to sit down in a hesitant and cajoling way. He ignored her, and she then began trying to physically drag him to a chair while he kicked and yelled. The father sat quietly and, occasionally, exchanged smirking glances with Nathan. He gave his wife several impatient looks as she began to get angry with the boy.

After waiting to see how this interaction would evolve, the therapist at this point commented that there were toys in a box that the parents could use to engage Nathan. The mother let go of the child to get a toy, then again pursued Nathan, who had scampered away from her reach. The father maintained his amused silence. By now, the therapist was postulating a strong alliance between father and son, which masked conflict between the parents. To test this assumption, the therapist commented that helping Nathan settle down seemed to be a two-person job and requested that the father help the mother. The father expressed annoyance at his wife's irritability with the boy and proceeded to get another toy from the box. What followed, was an astonishing sight, as the parents sat on the sofa, on either side of Nathan, and each simultaneously tried to get him interested in a different toy. Nathan was increasingly fidgety and agitated as the parents both talked at once to him, each seemingly oblivious to the other's attempt to engage his interest. Next, the therapist commented that the parents were each trying so hard to help the boy that neither seemed aware that they were each trying something different. They were asked to work together to get Nathan interested in one toy or another. The father managed to take leadership at this point, and the mother acquiesced immediately with a sigh of relief. Nathan began to pay attention at once as his father sounded quite firm.

After a few more suggestions to the parents that they tell Nathan what they expected, rather than asking and implying that they wanted *him* to choose, they managed to settle him at a table in the corner of the room with paper and crayons. He then proceeded to draw pictures for the next 20 minutes while the parents talked with the therapist. They glanced at their child frequently, and, after five minutes, began to express astonishment that he remained occupied. After ten minutes, his father solemnly announced that Nathan had never in his life been so quiet for so long. The therapist commented that it was clear the parents' discouragement had prevented them from realizing their competence to handle Nathan. She noted that Nathan clearly seemed to need both his parents to require the same thing from him at the same time, and to know that they agreed on what was best for him. The parents seemed subdued and bewildered, but nodded in agreement. They were given the task of taking Nathan to a restaurant that night, but only for dessert, and only for a half hour or less. They were given detailed instructions that Nathan should sit between the parents, and that his father should tell him what was expected, while his mother supported the father's instructions, as needed.

On the following day, the parents returned to excitedly report that they had contained Nathan in the restaurant the previous evening and had returned successfully with him for breakfast that morning. Anticipating resistance and possible regression in the face of such rapid change, the therapist suggested that they not expect things to be uphill from that point on. Also, they were encouraged not to attempt too much too soon in terms of more ambitious social ventures with Nathan. It was recommended that they eat in the room with Nathan that evening.* The parents then men-

---

* Various brands of family therapy employ the use of paradoxical techniques in the management of resistance, including the prevention of regression following sudden change. It is not possible here to elaborate the theoretical derivations of such techniques, but those readers interested in learning more about the modality of family therapy should pursue the literature.

tioned that the previous evening they had discussed their conviction that

Nathan's problems had a lot to do with long-standing conflict in their marriage. Nathan immediately became agitated at this point, and the parents were again give the task of containing him, which they accomplished fairly easily.

During the remainder of the second session and the following four sessions, the parents were repeatedly asked to work on the task of controlling Nathan. His father was asked to take leadership in giving clear directions to Nathan, and his mother was asked to give him affectionate approval of controlled behvior. Thus, each parent was afforded a chance to move out of the polarized and dysfunctional behaviors previously attempted with the boy. Instead of the father's being the "good guy," who pampered and infantilized his son, and the mother the ogre who angrily and ineffectively controlled him, each parent moved to a firm, warm, middle-of-the-road position.

In the last half of the last two sessions, the parents were encouraged to discuss marital problems which had gone unexpressed and unresolved in the face of their focus on Nathan's problems. Nathan became increasingly manageable in and out of the sessions.

The family was eating comfortably in restaurants by the end of the ten-day period. While it was clear that Nathan was a highly energetic, well coordinated, restless child, he responded quite well to firmness and clarity of expectations from his parents. Since his appetite had returned and symptoms improved during the period without medication, it was recommended that he not continue on the Ritalin.

A further recommendation was that Nathan be enrolled in a regular kindergarten in the fall, so the school personnel could observe his capacity to interact and learn with other normal youngsters. It was recognized that, given his intense nature, the school might wish to employ adjunctive services if he had difficulty in the future. For the present time, however, we felt that given the flexibility and progress Nathan had demonstrated during only a ten-day period, he deserved the chance to test his resources in a class with children whose potential more clearly approximated his rather than the retarded class he had experienced to date. The parents were encouraged to seek further family therapy at a later date if they felt the need.

Conclusion

This case and other similar successes with hyperactive children and their parents has led this therapist to conclude that the degree of intensity and the frequency of symptomatology in hyperactive children is very much related to the need of the system to support such symptoms. It is common enough that parents experiencing problems in their intimate relationship talk about their problems through their children. It follows, that with hyperactive children, it is the hyperactivity that would become the focus of these struggles. It must be assumed that the child who selects the symptoms that are usually associated with hyperactivity, as a way of communicating about stresses in the family, is probably biologically predisposed to this choice. The same statement could be made about children who choose some other psychosomatic symptom—and give up the symptom suddenly when the dysfunctional sequence of interaction in the family is interrupted. We consider the notion of dysfunctional sequencing to be primary—and consider that any *effective* modality has, whether deliberately or unwittingly, interrupted such a sequence. It should be stated that, at times, the dysfunctional sequence includes school personnel as well as parents. Thus, structural family therapists frequently study the school as well as the family in assessing a system which includes a symptomatic child.

To date, family therapy has received less attention than other modalities by those authorities interested in hyperactive children. We predict that professionals will increasingly discover and employ family therapy, particularly structural family therapy. It is efficient and effective.

References

CANTWELL, D. P. *The Hyperactive Child*. New York: Spectrum Publications, Inc., 1975.

CANTWELL, D. P. Psychiatric illness in the families of hyperactive children. *Arch. Gen. Psychiat.* 1972, 27:414-417.

FEIGHNER, A. C. and FEIGHNER, J. P. Multimodality treatment of the hyperkinetic child. *Amer. J. of Psychiat.* 1974, 131:459-463.

MINUCHIN, S. *Families and Family Therapy*. Cambridge, Mass.: Harvard University Press, 1974.

NEY, P. G. Four types of hyperkinesis. *Canadian Psychiatric Assoc. J.* 1974, 19: 543-550.

ROSS, D. M. and ROSS, S. A. *Hyperactivity*. New York: John Wiley & Sons, 1976.

SAFER, D. J. and ALLEN, R. P. *Hyperactive Children*. Baltimore: University Park Press, 1976.

SCHMITT, B. D., MARTIN, H. P., NELLHAUS, G., CRAVENS, J., CAMP, B. W., and JORDAN, K. The hyperactive child. *Clin. Pediat.* 1973, 12:154-169.

SCHRAG, P. and DIVOKY, D. *The Myth of the Hyperactive Child*. New York: Harper & Row, 1973.

STEWART, M. A. and OLDS, S. W. *Raising a Hyperactive Child*. New York: Harper & Row, 1973.

THOMAS, A., CHESS, S., and BIRCH, H. G. *Temperament and Behavior Disorders in Children*. New York: New York University Press, 1968.

WELNER, Z., WELNER, A., STEWART, M., PALKES, H., and WISH, E. A controlled study of siblings of hyperactive children. *J. Nerv. Ment. Dis.* 1977, 165:110-177.

CHAPTER 8

Diet Management

The major statement by Feingold (1975) concerning diet as a cause of hyperactivity has provoked an outpouring of pro and con reactions. Parent groups have been organized and there is now a national organization, The Feingold Association of the USA, committed to undertaking research and assisting parents in the area of diet management of hyperactivity.

Exactly how foods and food additives influence behavior is not always clear. In some instances, researchers are concerned with allergic responses; while in other cases, the food additives are thought to function as drugs, affecting neurological functioning so as to precipitate hyperactive responses.

The proponents of a "diet viewpoint," see it as an efficient and parsimonious solution to a behavior pattern that frustrates the child, his family, and teachers and is at best only manageable by interventions. As Wunderlich stated:

Many hyperkinetic children are allergic children by virtue of clinical history or by physical examination of the nasal mucous membranes. It is wise to remember that oranges, chocolate, egg, wheat, or milk can be directly responsible for hyperactive behavior. There is nothing more tragic than the untreated allergic hyperactive, for proper allergic management will often result in disappearance of the hyperactivity! (Wunderlich, 1970, pp. 300-301.)

The greatest support for diet management comes from parents who often maintain that they have seen remarkable behavior changes in their children as a result. Viewing diet as a major cause of hyperactivity is also reassuring to parents who may have felt that they had some part in causing the condition in their child. The scientific literature is considerably more conservative on the subject of diet management, evidencing mixed findings. As reviewed in the introductory chapter, there are supportive studies (Conners et al., 1976; Cook and Woodhill, 1976; Brenner, 1977), but there are also negative and mixed reports (Harley et al., 1978; Williams et al., 1978; Mattes and Gittelman-Klein, 1978).

Tryphonus, and Trites (1979) believed that food allergies are most closely associated with hyperactive children's exhibiting evidence of learning disabilities and minimal brain dysfunction. They also pointed out that the relationship of behavior to food allergies can be complex, as in the case of a person with weak sensitivity to a number of foods who may consume many of those foods within a short time period, and subsequently develop allergic symptoms.

Even when food factors are identified as probable contributors to hyperactivity, diet management can be very demanding and problematic for a family. The additives in many foods are inadequately labeled. Seemingly small violations of the diet will reportedly precipitate a renewal of the hyperactive behavior. Proponents of the Feingold diet are quick to point out that there is no such thing as a "partial diet." The burden of purchasing and preparing the food may be excessive for parents, raising the question of the "cure" possibly being worse than the "disease," in terms of the broader effects on the family.

In any event, hyperactivity viewed as an allergic or food-based neurological reaction needs to be taken seriously. The statement by Trites et al., in this chapter, that they have found 20 percent of hyperactive children to respond favorably to diet management, underscores the potential usefulness of diet study and control.

The three cases being presented illustrate the kinds of rationale and positive effects supportive of diet management. The reader should be reminded of the fact that *successful* cases studies were solicited for this book, and that the extent to which hyperactivity is related to and can be controlled by diet remains controversial.

References

BRENNER, A. A study of the efficacy of the Feingold diet on hyperkinetic children: Some favorable personal observations. *Clin. Pediat.* 1977, 16:652-656.

CONNERS, C. K., GOYETTE, C., SOUTHWICK, D., LEES, J., and ANDROLUNIS, P. Food additives and hyperkinesis: A controlled double-blind experiment. *Pediatrics* 1976, 58:154-166.

COOK, P. S., and WOODHILL, J. The Feingold dietary treatment of the hyperkinetic syndrome. *Med. J. Australia* 1976, 2:85-90.

FEINGOLD, B. F. *Why Your Child Is Hyperactive.* New York: Random House, 1975.

HARLEY, J. P., RAY, R. S., TOMASI, L., EICHMAN, P. L., MATHEWS, C. G., CHUN, R., CLEELAND, C. S., and TRAISMAN, E. Hyperkinesis and food additives: Testing the Feingold hypothesis. *Pediatrics* 1978, 61:818-828.

MATTES, J., and GITTELMAN-KLEIN, R. A crossover study of artificial food colorings in a hyperkinetic child. *Amer. J. Psychiat.* 1978, 135:987-988.

TRYPHONUS, H., and TRITES, R. Food allergy in children with hyperactivity, learning disabilities and/or minimal brain dysfunction. *Annals of Allergy* 1979, 42:22-27.

WILLIAMS, J. I., CRAM, D. M., TAUSIG, F. T., and WEBSTER, E. Relative effects of drugs and diet on hyperactive behaviors: An experimental study. *Pediatrics* 1978, 61:811-817.

WUNDERLICH, R. C. *Kids, Brains, and Learning.* St. Petersburg: Johnny Reads, 1970.

CASE STUDY #19. DIET MANAGEMENT WITH AN ELEVEN-YEAR-OLD BOY

Jeanne Mayo

Current Problem

Scott is an eleven-year-old, fifth grade boy who exhibits a variety of behavioral problems at home and at school. The teacher described him as physically overactive, aggressive, hostile, irritable, and easily frustrated. She reports that he talks back to authority figures, cries easily, and is generally disruptive in the classroom. He has poor concentration, short attention span, and difficulties in gross motor coordination. He compulsively touches everyone and everything. The teacher says he cannot easily be diverted from an action, and his tolerance for failure is low. He has difficulty in organizing and completing his school work; assignments are forgotten or handed in late. Scott's reading skills are poor. He seems to daydream and forgets instructions given by the teacher. He constantly defends his behavior. Verbal reprimands by the teacher are necessitated frequently. Scott has few friends and relationships with other children are difficult, with negative reactions.

Background Information

Scott was a full-term baby and pregnancy was normal. His one sibling, a girl, is three years younger than he. The parents are both professionals. Scott was an active, happy baby. His parents reported that his constant rooting in the crib caused the tip of his nose to be rubbed raw. Scott seemed to enjoy being with people and was very affectionate, as well as physically strong, outgoing, and curious.

Scott walked at approximately 11 months and spoke in discernable phrases by two years of age. He was toilet trained by two years of age. He was administered the Stanford Binet at age 2½ and obtained an IQ score of 130.

At age four, Scott was enrolled in a pre-school program so that he could be with other children. The teacher complained to his parents that Scott could not sit still during story time, was disruptive to the class, and could not keep his hands to himself.

At age five, Scott went into the school's kindergarten program. His academic progress was slow. Behavioral reports from his teacher were again poor. The teacher described him as an aggressive child who had poor concentration and a short attention span. His fine motor control was below average; printing, drawing, and coloring activities were poor and difficult.

In the first grade, Scott continued to experience problems in reading and printing. His difficulty in sitting still was reported by the teacher. She felt that ignoring the unacceptable behavior would discourage it. However, this approach did not improve Scott's behavior.

In the second grade, Scott was referred to the resource teacher for learning disability testing. The tests indicated visual and auditory perceptual problems. An achievement test was also administered in math and reading. Scott was found to be on grade level in mathematics. He scored two years below average in reading, however, and thereby, qualified for academic assistance from the resource room. He spent one hour a day in the resource room and one hour after school in a special reading class for children with reading problems.

His parents took Scott for medical examinations by the family pediatrician and an ophthalmologist. Both physicians agreed that Scott was hyperactive and suffered from visual perceptual problems. He was referred back to the resource teacher for therapy.

The second grade classroom teacher frequently reprimanded Scott verbally for disruptive behavior and seated him in the back of the room, separated from the rest of the class. This approach did not improve his academic or behavioral problems, in fact, Scott began to develop self-esteem problems. He would frequently come home from school crying, and tell his mother that he was dumb. He reported that the other children teased him and called him names on the way home from school. He was not allowed by the teacher to go on field trips with the class.

Six weeks into the third grade, Scott's parents were called to the school for a conference by the classroom teacher, the resource teacher, and the principal. The teacher reported that Scott was the "worst" child in the classroom. The aggressive, hostile, disruptive behavior had warranted a poor grade in conduct for the six-week period. The resource teacher's prognosis for his advancement in reading was poor. She suggested that Scott be placed on a behavior modifying medication so that he would not continue to be disruptive in the classroom. More comprehensive academic tutoring was discussed.

Intervention

The resource room provided a one-to-one situation that included remediation and reinforcement for academic progress. Scott's behavior and achievement showed improvement in the resource room, but this progress did not generalize into the classroom. The only additional intervention suggested by the resource teacher was medication. Scott's parents, however, learned about diet as a possible factor in causing hyperactivity and decided instead to begin a diet intervention program at home. The teachers were told that the child would receive additional help, but were not informed of the type of program so as to avoid the effect of suggestion. Scott was immediately placed on the Kaiser-Permanente Feingold diet (Appendix A as outlined by Dr. Benjamin Feingold, 1975). A daily diet diary of all foods eaten by Scott was kept by his mother for six weeks.

Each day the teacher and the parents assigned the child a conduct grade. The grade was then translated into a numerical score. The individual score of the parents and teacher were combined and averaged to yield one composite score for each day. The scoring system was as follows:

$$A = 100 \text{ percent} = \text{Excellent}$$
$$B = 75 \text{ percent} = \text{Good}$$
$$C = 50 \text{ percent} = \text{Average}$$
$$D = 25 \text{ percent} = \text{Below average}$$
$$E = 0 \text{ percent} = \text{Very poor}$$

The combined teacher and parent ratings were averaged for each 10-day time period when the child was on the diet. The 12 time periods, therefore, reflect data collected for 16 weeks (four months). There were, of course, days when the child went off the diet accidentally or on purpose, and these days cannot be considered *on-diet days*.

Since dietary infraction can cause an effect for three days after the infraction occurs, the *off-diet* rating includes the day of the dietary infraction plus the rating for the following two days. Therefore, the time periods for *on-diet* and *off-diet* averages are not the same. The *on-diet* ratings were averaged over a 10-day period (minus the infraction days) while the *off-diet* ratings averaged were over a three-day period. It should be noted that there were no dietary infractions for periods five, six, seven, and eight. The total is an average of the ratings over the sixteen weeks. The average behavioral rating for *on-diet* days was 65 percent while the average for *off-diet* days was 36 percent.

The on- and off-diet data is summarized in Table 1. All seven periods in which both on- and off-diet data were obtained, yielded higher ratings for the on-diet days. This result is associated with an exact binomial $p \leqslant 0.0078$.

The teacher called Scott's parents 10 days after the Feingold program was initiated, reporting a positive change in his behavior. The hostile and

TABLE 1

Average Behavioral Ratings for On- and Off-Diet Periods

	Average Behavioral Ratings	
10-Day Periods	On-Diet	Off-Diet
1	46%	8%
2	79%	25%
3	64%	58%
4	81%	42%
5	65%	—
6	70%	—
7	63%	—
8	63%	—
9	57%	42%
10	88%	42%
11	54%	25%
12	50%	—
TOTAL	65%	36%

Exact $p \leqslant 0.0078$

aggressive behavior had disappeared. Six weeks after the diet was begun, Scott received the first "G" (good) for a conduct grade on his report card. Further ratings of checks (satisfactory) had replaced minuses (unsatisfactory) in three areas: disciplines himself, responds promptly and willingly, and works and plays well with others. The following report card after six weeks showed that the G (good) in conduct had been maintained and the two remaining minuses had been changed to checks. The new checked areas were: uses time and materials effectively, and follows direction. These grades were maintained throughout the school year, with an exception of one six-week period.

Scott's parents removed him from the Feingold diet for a six-week period during the spring semester. Neither the teacher nor Scott was told of the change. Scott's conduct grade dropped to an unsatisfactory level. He received minuses again on three areas of conduct: disciplines himself, responds promptly and willingly, and works and plays well with others. Scott was returned to the diet for the next six-week period. All grades subsequently returned to satisfactory.

During the last month of the third grade, Scott was retested by the resource teacher for an assessment of visual perceptual problems. His scores were all normal. Group achievement test scores showed, however, that Scott was still below his level for reading. Language skill and arithmetic concepts were well above average. An individual intelligence test IQ score (WISC) was 125.

Scott was retested for the resource room at the beginning of grade four, but did not score the two years below level in reading that was required to qualify for help. During the year, he was moved from the low reading group in his class into the middle group and maintained a B average in reading. Scott received a consistent B average in conduct for the year. He received above average marks in the area of "works and plays well with others." Group-achievement test scores showed that Scott had accomplished a four-year increase in reading in one year and with this score was well above average.

Scott won second place out of 200 boys in the Cub Scout Olympics for his city and pitched a no-loss season on his Little League baseball team. He received an award at his piano recital for the "most progress made for a boy" over the year. He was elected president of his class.

Conclusion

Scott's pediatrician, teachers, and parents determined that Scott's behavior was affected by the synthetic additives in his diet. One prohibited food would lead to a negative behavioral reaction. The reaction would last for approximately three days. His teacher learned to recognize a negative reaction and encouraged Scott to control his behavior on his own. Two reactions were extreme, and the teacher called his mother to come and take Scott home. He remained home until the reaction was over.

Scott participated in the decision to try the Feingold diet. Once a positive response had been achieved, Scott adhered willingly to the program, because it made him feel better.

A placebo effect was considered when the diet was begun. However, the longer the positive response, the more doubtful was the placebo effect. It was suggested that the attention given Scott over a special diet could contribute to the positive change. Although, it was argued that Scott has received attention throughout all the treatments previous to the Feingold program. Mistakes were made over the initial six-week period, followed by a negative behavior reaction each time. Some mistakes were not discovered until a negative reaction was observed.

Although a positive behavior change was observed within weeks after beginning the Feingold diet, academic progress was much slower. In Scott's case, a dramatic change, especially in reading skills, occurred in approximately a period of one year, and progress subsequenlty continued.

Reference

FEINGOLD, B. *Why Your Child is Hyperactive.* New York: Random House, 1975.

CASE STUDY #20. DIET MANAGEMENT
WITH A SEVEN-YEAR-OLD BOY

Jeanne Mayo

Current Problem

Since he was four years old and until he was seven-years-old and placed on a diet management program, Sammy's behavior had shown a consistent pattern. He chattered continuously, but had difficulty completing sentences. He moved about constantly with jerky, bouncy movements, and compulsively touched other children. After having his thumb in his mouth, he would approach another child and run his hand up and down his arm. When in a store, he would rub the window glass in the same thoughtless manner. This type of behavior usually preceded a slow build-up of frustration until Sammy seemed to be worked into a frenzy.

He could not be diverted from an action and his behavior was usually unpredictable. Sammy expressed his frustration in the form of temper tantrums; his demands had to be met immediately even though at times he did not seem to know what it was that he wanted. Sammy cried easily and often. The mother reported that when Sammy experienced a negative behavioral reaction, he could not be easily calmed. He would scream and display hostile and aggressive behavior. He would curse adults and fight with other children, as well as impulsively attack his mother by hitting her or suddenly grabbing her hair. On one occasion, Sammy was bitten by the family dog after he attacked the pet. When physically injured, he did not scream nor cry; for example, he ignored the splinters in his hands that he got from trying to climb the backyard fence at home.

Sammy was unable to sit through a meal or television program. Sometimes he was unable to decide whether to play in the backyard or to watch television and would become frustrated. He encountered difficulty in unbuttoning his clothes and would become impatient and jerk the clothes off. His mother reported that Sammy experienced severe insomnia and enuresis.

In his early school experiences, Sammy demonstrated a short attention span, poor concentration, inability to complete his work, poor eye-hand motor coordination, difficulty in drawing or writing, and difficulty with playground activities. He was unable to sit through a school project, often ran about the classroom, and disturbed other children.

From these behaviors, it was evident that Sammy was a hyperactive child. It should be made clear, that although Sammy had some compulsive and repetitive behaviors, he was not considered to be autistic. He talked continuously, he did not rock, and generally had a warm relationship with his mother.

Background Information

Sammy was a full-term baby and there were no problems encountered during the pregnancy. His mother was 40 years old at the time of birth. His only siblings are much older than Sammy. The development of the two older children was reported as normal. His mother described Sammy as a very happy baby and said that he seldom cried, and seemed to enjoy being with people. Sammy never learned to crawl, but pushed himself up when he was nine months old and began walking. He began babbling when he was only a few months old and began speaking in discernable phrases when he was three. Sammy was a strong, active baby. Toilet training was difficult, but was accomplished by three years of age. However, Sammy continued to have accidents until he was seven years old and, if he was not reminded to go to the toilet, would put it off until it was too late.

At the age of five, Sammy entered a private pre-school program. He had to be forced to enter the classroom each day and stayed close to the teacher throughout the school day. The teacher reported that Sammy could not be disciplined; he cried, and seemed unhappy. Sammy was slow in fine motor skills; drawing was difficult for him. He was, however, successful at memorization and oral recitation.

The teacher suggested that the child's physician be contacted concerning Sammy's learning and behavioral problems. Sammy was placed on Ritalin, but experienced further deterioration in behavior. He refused to eat and the insomnia became worse; therefore, the Ritalin was discontinued. At the end of the pre-school program, Sammy was six years old and was tested by a school psychologist. He was given Screening Language and Learning Assessment for Training (SSLAT).

The scores on the SSLAT were as follows:

Comprehension	3 years, 9 months
Expressiveness	4 years, 3 months
Articulation	6 years, 1 month
Visual-memory	3 years, 0 months
Auditory-memory	3 years, 6 months
Ability to trace or follow a pattern	3 years, 9 months

Sammy obtained an I.Q. score of 68 on the Stanford Binet Intelligence Test. A diagnosis of mental retardation was made on the basis of these tests scores.

Sammy entered the first grade in the public schools, but had to be forced to go into the classroom each day and cried frequently. Because of his general immaturity, Sammy was put back in a kindergarten class. The teacher indicated that Sammy could do his class work and was anxious to please her, but talked excessively and was generally disruptive in the classroom. On the basis of Sammy's continuing problems, he was placed in a special education kindergarten. The purpose of this class was to train children who had been diagnosed with minimal brain dysfunction.

Sammy continued in this class but was referred to a neurological clinic for further testing and diagnosis. He was examined by both a neurologist and a psychologist. His EEG was normal, but on the basis of the neurological examination, he was diagnosed as having brain dysfunction. The Wechsler Intelligence Scale for children yielded an IQ score of 68. The clinic suggested that Sammy be trained in a special program and Ritalin was again prescribed for his learning and behavioral problems. Sammy was given a sedative while at the clinic and on the way home became agitated and tried to break the glass in the windows of the car.

Since Ritalin had not been effective previously, and the sedative had agitated the child, the parents felt that the medication should not be tried again. Sammy's mother decided to try the Feingold diet (Feingold, 1975) and contacted the local Feingold Association. The parents were concerned about the diagnosis of mental retardation, since they had seen no evidence of mental retardation at home. His mother felt that the I.Q. scores might have been adversely affected by Sammy's hyperactive behavior. Therefore, she felt that further testing needed to be done only after Sammy's behavior was under control.

Intervention

Sammy was participating in an individualized learning program which employed behavior modification techniques. Since the program was not fully effective, however, his parents felt that other alternatives needed to be explored. They decided to place Sammy on the Feingold diet. The Feingold Program for hyperactive children is a selective buying program which eliminates colors, preservatives, and natural salicylates from the child's diet. (Appendix A) The parents began this diet with the cooperation of the teacher. A parent counselor from the Feingold Association assisted the family by calling once a week to answer questions and give encouragement. Sammy's mother kept a diet diary and noted everything he ate. In this way, she could determine which foods and chemicals Sammy could not tolerate. At school, the teacher began to reward Sammy with trinkets rather than candy. Therefore, Sammy was on the diet both at home and at school.

Three weeks after the Feingold Program was initiated, improvement was noted both at home and at school. At home, Sammy appeared to be much calmer; he could now sleep all night and enuresis was gone. Within three weeks after the diet was begun, the teacher reported that Sammy could sit quietly and listen in the reading circle. In addition, his interactions with other children at school improved.

At the end of the school year, Sammy was seven years old and his report card showed improvement in many areas. He received a grade of A+ in the following conduct area: shows respect for others and willingness to correct work. He also showed improvement in the following areas: obedience, follows directions, works independently, and practices self-discipline. The group achievement scores yielded the following results: reading 1.2 (first grade, 2 months), math (pre-kindergarten—7 months), and spelling (pre-kindergarten—5 months). Although these tests scores were not on grade level for Sammy's age at that time, it is important to remember that at the end of the school year, he had just finished the kindergarten level.

The next year, Sammy entered the first grade and continued to receive help in special education. His behavior and academic work continued to improve during the year. At the end of the first grade, Sammy was eight years old and, although he was not performing at an eight-year level, he was performing up to his grade level.

His test scores at the end of the first grade were as follows:

Reading	1.9 (first grade, 9 months)
Math	2.2 (second grade, 2 months)
Spelling	1.6 (first grade, 6 months)

As can be seen from these scores, Sammy made considerable progress in that year. His report card yielded the following grades:

Handwriting	B+
Language	A+
Spelling	A
Reading	A
Arithmetic	B

He continued to make progress in his conduct and behavior. Sammy received a grade of A+ (above average) in the following areas: attention, makes good use of time, habits, and follows directions. These areas are particularly important since he had received a minus grade on these the previous year.

Conclusion

Sammy's achievement scores indicate that he made the equivalent of seven months' progress in reading, and over three years' progress in math and spelling in one year. It appears that it would be impossible for a mentally retarded child to make this much progress in one year. With continued improvement, Sammy should eventually be on grade level and be able to enter a regular class. His behavior at home and school continues to improve. Sammy has continued to stay on the diet and his academic and behavioral progress are being followed.

Reference

FEINGOLD, B. *Why Your Child is Hyperactive.* New York: Random House, 1975.

APPENDIX A

THE FEINGOLD DIET

The Kaiser-Permanente (K-P) or Feingold Diet is a selective buying program, originally developed by Dr. Benjamin F. Feingold, Professor Emeritus, Department of Allergy, Kaiser-Permanente Medical Center, and author of *Why Your Child Is Hyperactive.*

On this program, the basic diet of the child is not necessarily changed. However, only the approved foods, by brand names, are used. Chemical additives such as synthetic colors, synthetic flavors, BHA/BHT (anti-oxidants), and natural salicyclates are eliminated. The natural salicylates are almonds, apples, apricots, tomatoes, cucumbers, berries, cherries, currant, grapes, oranges, peaches, and plums. Natural additives such as salt, spices, herbs, and vinegar are allowed. Refined carbohydrates are limited depending upon individual tolerances.

After a positive response has been observed on the K-P diet, each of the natural salicylates is returned to the child's diet individually, and tested for a negative reaction.

A positive response in behavior should be observed within a six-week period after beginning the diet. This response should not be expected if a child is also on behavior modifying drugs. Ingestion of a prohibited food by the child, after a positive change in behavior is accomplished, will cause a negative behavior reaction to occur. A discernable negative change in behavior or learning usually will occur within several hours after the food is consumed. The reaction can last for approximately three days; thus a bite on Monday and another Thursday can negate the entire week. Therefore, the diet must be adhered to 100 percent.

Fumes, aromas, and products applied topically can have similar effect. Therefore, the child must also avoid: glue, paint, hand lotion, perfumes, hair sprays, ink on the skin, "scratch and sniff notebooks," colored chalk, air freshners, scented candles, colored and flavored medications, colored toothpaste, etc.

CASE STUDY #21. TREATMENT OF HYPERACTVITY IN A CHILD WITH ALLERGIES TO FOODS*

Ronald L. Trites, Helen Tryphonas, and Bruce Ferguson

There is increasing evidence that hyperactivity in children is a final common result from a variety of etiological factors. Among these are neurological complications following prenatal or perinatal trauma (Minde et al., 1968); maternal smoking during pregnancy (Dawson et al., 1976); exposure to metals such as lead (David, 1974); fluorescent lights (Arehart-Teichel, 1974); stress and genetic transmission (Waldrop and Halverson, 1971); and artificial food additives such as colors, flavors, and preservatives (Feingold, 1975). In addition, a variety of neuropsychological manifestations in children are thought to be caused by adverse allergic reactions to inhalants and foods. Symptoms of irritability, fatigue, hyperactivity, or severe mental depression diminish or disappear following elimination of certain foods from the child's diet (Clarke, 1950).

Follow-up studies have shown that hyperactive children are at high risk for school drop-out, psychiatric problems, abuse of drugs, alcoholism, and criminality (Barcai, 1974; Blouin et al., in press; Goodwin et al., 1975). These discouraging results are mainly due to the fact that hyperactive children with heterogenous etiologies have been grouped together and often administered only one mode of treatment consisting of stimulant drugs. Perhaps the long term results would be more encouraging if there were rationale for treatment, and treatment choice were more closely matched with a given etiology.

In the Neuropsychology Laboratory at the Royal Ottawa Hospital, a large long-term investigation of hyperactivity is underway. The purpose of

* This study was supported primarily by Grant 606-1237-44 from the Research Programs Directorate, Health and Welfare Canada.

such a study is to develop a rationale for the treatment of hyperactivity. In this study, hyperactive children are intensively investigated on a variety of neuropsychological, personality, neurological, psychophysiological, biochemical, and immunological parameters in an attempt to carefully subgroup the children's conditions. A variety of treatments is then systematically tried on each subgroup, including stimulant drug, behavioral therapy, and elimination diet. Children in each subgroup are then followed over a three-year period, at the end of which an attempt is being made to match the most effective treatment with the particular subgroup of hyperactive children.

We are presently investigating the possible association of food to hyperactivity in specific subgroups of hyperactive children in ways other than the adverse reactions to artificial food additives theory first described by Feingold (1975) and carefully studied by Conners et al. (1976). For example, it is found that approximately two-thirds of the hyperactive children tested have elevated levels of specific reaginic (IgE) antibody to one or more of 42 different food extracts tested by the radioallergosorbent test RAST (Tryphonas & Trites, Note 1). Phadebas RAST Kits (Pharmacia Laboratories; Montreal, Quebec) are used to determine serum IgE antibodies directed against specific food allergens (Chau et al., 1976; Haddad and Korotzer, 1972). Radioactivity in the test and control tubes is measured using a Beckman's Y-counter. RAST scores (0-4) are based on a serially diluted reference serum supplied by Pharmacia. A score of one or greater is considered to be positive.

The validity of the RAST results is further investigated in a doubleblind cross-over study. During this study, half of the children are instructed to follow a treatment diet which eliminates all foods that evidence a positive RAST result for a period of three weeks. The treatment diet is followed by a placebo diet for the same duration. The placebo diet is designed to exclude foods equal in number and nutritionally equivalent to those included in the treatment diet, but having negative RAST results. For the other half of the children, the order of the diets is reversed. The following case report focuses on a child belonging to this specific subgroup of hyperactive children.

Daniel

Current Problem and Background Information

Daniel was a six-year, seven-month-old male, enrolled in a transition class, between kindergarten and grade one. The product of a full-term pregnancy, he weighed 7 lbs. 13 oz. at birth. There were no reported complications. His milestones were normal and he suffered nothing but the usual childhood illnesses. However, at the age of approximately one year, Daniel's parents became concerned about his behavior, particularly his increasing activity, aggressiveness toward his younger brother, and severe temper tantrums which occurred several times a day. These problems gradually increased to the extent that he could no longer be left unsupervised.

At the age of five years and 10 months, Daniel received a neuropsychological examination, which consisted of various language, perceptual, IQ, and academic achievement tests, along with a detailed standardized motor and sensory examination (Trites, 1978). He scored a Verbal IQ of 104, Performance IQ of 103, and a Full Scale IQ of 104 on the Wechsler Intelligence Scale for Children. Academic achievement testing indicated that reading, spelling, and arithmetic skills were at the beginning grade-one level. Motor and sensory functions were normal. Teachers' ratings on the Conners Rating Scale (Conners, 1969) substantiated the parents' ratings and clinical judgment that this was a highly hyperactive youngster who was physically well developed, well coordinated, and possessed at least average learning potential. He was then placed on a trial of Methylphenidate (Ritalin), 15 mg t.i.d. The parents and teacher reported that they noticed no beneficial effects of the drug; in fact, he appeared to be more unmanageable while on it.

Intervention

As part of the extensive baseline evaluations, Daniel was examined for the presence of allergies to foods. His parents were carefully instructed and a complete three-week food diary was obtained. From the diary, a list of 42 foods most commonly consumed by the child was obtained and the RAST test was performed. Clinically significant levels of specific reaginic antibody were detected to oats and rye, with a RAST score of one for each of the foods.

In addition, information pertaining to allergies in the child and his family (siblings, parents, and grandparents) was obtained by directly interviewing the patient and his parents via an itemizing allergy questionnaire. Daniel's history did not reveal the presence of any allergies. However, a review of the family history of allergy disclosed that his maternal grandmother suffered from severe asthma since she was five years old. At the age of 22 years, asthma became gradually milder, giving way to hayfever. The latter persists to date, at the age of 75. Daniel's mother also developed severe hayfever at the age of 15. This condition persists to date, but in a mild form. Furthermore, Daniel's mother and grandmother suffered from a mild sporadic eczema.

Daniel was rated by his parents and teacher (Conners parent and teacher Questionnaires) prior to being placed on the three-week treatment elimination diet which excluded all foods containing oats and rye diet. He was also reassessed before being placed on the three-week placebo diet, during which an equal number of foods to which he did not show an allergic reaction were removed systematically from his diet, in order to measure placebo effects. In addition, the child was rated daily during the treatment and

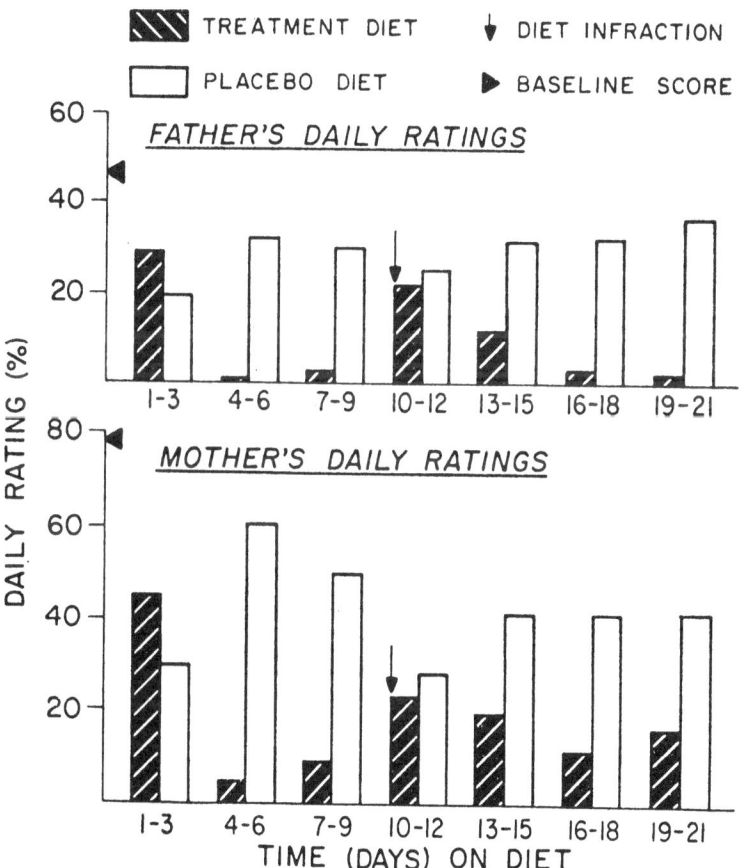

FIG. 1. Parent Daily Ratings (%) of Hyperactivity (Conners Parent Questionnaire) for Treatment and Placebo Diets.

placebo diets independently by his mother and father, using the short form of the Conners Parent Rating Scale (Conners, 1970). Furthermore, the parents were instructed to review with Daniel all of the foods he had eaten and list any infractions of the diet daily.

Considering the mother's ratings first, it can be seen from Figure 1 that the baseline rating of hyperactivity which she assigned to Daniel was almost 80 percent on the Conners Scale. Under both elimination and placebo diet phases, the ratings tended to be diminished as compared to baseline. However, there was clear evidence of a substantial beneficial effect when foods to which Daniel was considered to be allergic, (the cross-hatched bars) were eliminated from his diet. During day 10, this youngster inadvertently went off his diet and ratings of hyperactivity increased, followed by a gradual decrease once again of levels of hyperactivity on succeeding days.

Baseline levels of the father's independent ratings were lower than the mother's analogous ratings. It is, in our experience, typical for fathers to rate their children as somewhat less hyperactive than mothers. However, from the father's ratings there was also significant diet treatment effect. In fact, in the three-day periods 4 to 6 and 7 to 9, Daniel's behavior had dramatically improved, as was the case with the mother's ratings. The father also reported an increase in hyperactivity in the three-day period (days 10 to 12) when the child inadvertently went off the diet. This was followed once again by an improvement in behavior in the subsequent three-day periods.

Conclusions

The study of Daniel presents support for a diet management position with selected children. We have found that approximately 20 percent of hyperactive children show a substantial improvement on an elimination diet, controlling for specific foods to which the child is allergic. We are currently monitoring the progress of hyperactive children with food allergies maintained on an elimination diet, since this appears to be a promising treatment approach for some of these children.

Reference Note

1. TRYPHONAS, H. and TRITES, R. L. *Food Allergy in Children with Hyperactivity, Learning Disabilities and/or Minimal Brain Dysfunction.* Manuscript in preparation, 1979.

References

AREHART-TEICHEL. Hoan school lights and problem pupils. *Science News* 1974, 105: 258-259.

Barcai, Avner. A precursor of delinquency: The hyperkinetic disorder of childhood. *Psychiatric Quarterly* 1974, 48:387-399.

Blouin, A. G. A., Bornstein, R. A., and Trites, R. L. Teenage alcohol abuse among hyperactive children: A five-year follow-up study. *J. Pediatric Psychol.* In press.

Chua, Y. Y., Bremmer, K., Dakdawalla, N., Llobet, J. K., Kokuba, H. L., and Orange, R. P. In vivo and in vitro correlates of food allergy. *J. Allergy and Clin. Immunol.* 1976, 58(2):299-307.

Clarke, T. W. The relation of allergy to character problems in children: A survey. *Psychiatric Quarterly* 1950, 24:21-38.

Conner, C. K. A teacher rating scale for use in studies with children. *Amer. J. Psychiat.* 1969, 126:884-888.

Conners, C. K., Goyette, C. H., Southwick, D. A., Less, J. M., and Andrulonis, P. A. Food additives and hyperkinesis: A controlled double-blind experiment. *Pediatrics* 1976, 58:154-164.

Conners, C. K. Symptom patterns in hyperkinetic, neurotic, and normal children. *Child Devel.* 1970, 41:667-682.

David, O. J. Association between lower level lead concentration and hyperactivity in children. *Environmental Health Perspectives* 1974, 7:17-25.

Dawson, R., Nanson, J. L., and McWatters, M. A. Hyperkinesis and maternal smoking. *Canadian Psychiat. Assoc. J.* 1976, 20:183-187.

Feingold, Ben F. *Why Your Child is Hyperactive.* New York: Random House, 1975.

Goodwin, D. W., Schulsinger, F., Hermansen, L., Guze, S. B., and Winokur, G. *J. Nerv. Ment. Dis.* 1975, 16:349-353.

Haddad, Z. H., and Korotzer, J. L. Immediate hypersensitivity reactions to food antigens. *J. Allergy and Clin. Immunol.* 1972, 49, (4):210-218.

Minde, K., Webb, C., and Sykes, D. Studies on the hyperactive child: VI prenatal and perinatal factors associated with hyperactivity. *Dev. Med. and Child Neurol.* 1968, 10:355-363.

Trites, R. L. *Neuropsychological Test Manual.* Montreal: Ronalds Federated, 1978.

Waldrop, M., and Halverson, C. F. Minor physical anomalies and hyperactive behavior in your children. In Hellmuth, J. (ed.), *Exceptional Infant*, Volume II. New York: Brunner/Mazel, 1971, pp. 343-389.

Part III
MEASUREMENT, DIAGNOSIS, AND INTERVENTION

CHAPTER 9

A Review and Appraisal of Instruments Assessing Hyperactivity in Children

JOHN P. POGGIO AND
NEIL J. SALKIND

Since the early 1960's, hyperactivity in children has received increased attention from psychologists, physicians, and educators. Theoretical models (Ross and Ross, 1976; Fine, 1977), extensive basic research, and a variety of treatment programs now exist, which document both the attention and intentions paid to this topic. However, the basic step toward treatment or remediation, the provision of adequate assessment procedures, has not yet been fully accomplished.

Although conceptual definitions are useful when formulating a theoretical perspective, it is the operational definition that becomes paramount when attempts are made at designing research or treatment programs. In spite of the wide breadth of research being conducted, it is still relatively unclear how effective and powerful available instruments are in the assessment of activity level, both from an applied and a theoretical perspective (Salkind and Poggio, 1975, 1977; Sandoval, 1977). The laxity with which hyper-

---

* This article appeared in *Learning Disabilities Quarterly* and is being reproduced here by permission of the authors and the publisher.

activity has been "operationally" defined, presents a background against which the results of reported research are ambiguous, nonspecific, and lacking in generalizability. It appears that a premium has been placed on recording the outcomes of assessment techniques, rather than on the adequacy of the definition of hyperactivity, and the characteristics of the assessment devices themselves.

The purpose of this chapter is to offer a critical appraisal of a selected group of instruments commonly used to assess activity level (and in particular hyperactivity) in young children. The review is limited to observational types of instruments, since retrospective, narrative, and mechanical procedures are (1) less frequently used in applied situations; (2) fewer in number; and (3) especially in the case of mechanical instruments, expensive to construct or purchase, inconvenient to use, and often too invasive to obtain an accurate estimate of the behavior independent of the method.

This review of existing instrumentation is by no means all inclusive; there is a host of other variables, such as willingness to seek stimulation, for example, that are theoretically related to hyperactivity. Indeed, the measurement of these variables might provide more information about the nature of hyperactivity than a broad general approach to the condition itself. The devices included in this review were chosen because they appear to be the most popularly used observational instruments, reported in the literature. However, there are undoubtedly many other instruments that purport to measure "hyperactivity" (and activity level), and all should be weighed independently for their theoretical and psychometric credibility.

The first part of this chapter contains a description of some of the problems encountered in the assessment of hyperactivity, as well as a discussion of frequently used scales; in terms of their development, purpose and format, reliability, validity, and general useability. A summary of these instruments and their different characteristics is presented in Table 1. The second part of this chapter contains an annotated bibliography of other related scales and instruments that are relatively new to the field, or are in the process of being developed. Finally, the last part of the chapter contains some conclusions and recommendations for future instrument design and development.

The Problem of Definition

Few attempts have been made at defining hyperactivity, without the advantage of a sound empirical base. There is danger in defining hyperactivity without empirical referents, however, since the definition of different types of activity has a direct influence on the measurement and evaluation procedures used to assess the behaviors. The most popular practice (and perhaps the one most lacking in construct validity) is to use synonyms that reflect behaviors of the hyperactive child, but do not advance any one definition. In fact, Keogh (1971) has commented that "most investigators focus on the symptomatology of the condition without defining the construct" (p. 102).

Adding confusion to the nebulous issue of definition, the term hyperactive is also used as a synonym for such terms as hyperkinetic, short attention span, mood fluctuation, impulsivity, restlessness, distractibility, overactivity, hypermotility neurosis, minimal brain dysfunction, postencephaltic behavior disorder, and organic driveness. Terminology that is equally characteristic and descriptive of other childhood difficulties is also frequently employed in describing the hyperactive chlid: e.g., negativism, poor judgment, and irritability (Delong, 1972). At best, such descriptors often have only content or face validity, allowing for convenient but far less exact definition.

There appears to be a widespread practice of defining hyperactivity, and operating within the sphere of the hyperactive child, using techniques and/or instruments that often lack a direct substantial link to any theoretical construct. The task of subdividing the component parts of the concept of hyperactivity into more manageable and testable units, relating both theory and assessment procedures to one another, is both a major task and a goal in the search for credible measurement techniques.

Lack of Standardization

Another fundamental problem in the measurement of activity level, is that standards or norms for what constitutes the range and/or intensity of activity level are nonexistent. All too often, standards are presented in clinical terms that maximize the potential for a subjective interpretation of a behavior. For example, Cromwell et al. (1963) indicated that "superactivity" may be illusory or unreal, since estimates of another individual's activity level are often affected by and interpreted in light of a variety of interrelated factors.

Although normative data have not been reported, several investigators imply the existence of some normal level of activity functioning in their definitions. For example, Chess (1959) viewed the hyperactive child as "one who carries out activities at a higher rate of speed than the average child, or is constantly in motion, or both" (p. 2379). Werry (1968), and

Simpson and Nelson (1974) have made similar inferences. Eisenberg (1966) also referred to hyperactivity in childhood as motor activity in excess of the normal range for the child's age and sex. Schmitt et al. (1973) defined a hyperactive child as one whose motor activity is excessive for his/her mental age and sex. Excessive activity is said to exist when several people complain about it.

Such attempts at definition are insufficient, and are more confusing and detrimental than beneficial. It seems that establishing the boundaries of activity level more often results as a by-product of experimental research of the phenomenon itself, rather than research that quantitatively establishes norms. It is conceivable that the absence of standardized norms can result in classifications of children as "hyperactive, normal, or hypoactive," all of whom are in fact quite "normal," relative to the behavior "hyperactive." Efforts should be undertaken to establish reliable norms characterizing ranges of activity levels.

Multidimensionality of Activity Level

In describing four methods of measuring activity level (direct visual observation, free space traversal, fidgeometric, and kinometric), Cromwell et al. (1963) point out how different assessment techniques may ignore important intra-individual characteristics related to different types of activity. For example, direct visual observation utilizes frequency as the parameter that identifies a behavior, whereas a fidgeometric technique, such as the ballistograph, measures the intensity with which the subject jars or vibrates the platform on which he or she is placed. While both techniques indicate that activity is taking place, the two types of activity might be relatively independent of each other.

To further document this multidimensional structure, McConnell and Cromwell (1964) discuss activity level as the lower bound of hyperactivity, yet their comparison between scores on the *Child Rating Scale* (CRS), which includes those behavioral terms most often used in describing the syndrome, and the ballistograph, found the two to be unrelated. Schulman et al. (1965) also failed to find a statistically significant relationship between activity level, as measured by the actometer and other behavioral indices that they examined. Research by Conrad and Dusell (1967) also indicated a discrepancy between the experimental claim of significant results and practitioners' clinical impressions of the effectiveness of amphetamines on hyperactive behavior.

The lack of established validity, as well as those studies which found no relationship using different techniques, strongly suggests the existence of more than one type of activity level or form of hyperactivity. In summarizing earlier research, Cromwell et al. (1963) point out that "information available is sufficient to suggest that activity level should not be viewed as a single or homogeneous phenomenon" (p. 635). Reed (1947) expressed similar thoughts earlier, "what data we have, points to more than one type, or at least more than one aspect of activity" (p. 395). Morgan and Stellar (1950) defined three bipolar descriptors of activity level: locomotor versus diffuse, relevant versus irrelevant, and goal directed versus nongoal directed. In the development of a movement recording device, Bell (1968) concluded that more than one type of activity exists, and that "components and manifestations of activity in different measurement situations should be studied, rather than activity as a unitary invariant function" (p. 303). Pope and Pope (1969) suggested that a number of different levels or types of activity are of importance, and that any attempt at defining hyperactivity should take into account both the amount of activity and the focus and direction. More recently, Loo and Wenar (1971) have delineated three different types of activity: activity level as the quantitative amount of motoric movements, motor inhibition as the degree of ability to inhibit motor impulses, and impulsivity as the lack of self-control in modes other than motoric.

From these studies, one concludes that activity level is being conceptualized in numerous ways, and a number of different types or levels of activity have indeed been identified. The result has been that different techniques and instruments have focused on specific subclasses or categories of activity level resulting in greater confusion, inconsistent findings, and a myopic view of the behavior.

The development of a taxonomy of activity levels would be useful, since such a taxonomy should stress the classification of different types of activity levels and modes of hyperactivity, thus providing a more clearly defined conceptual base. Investigations could be undertaken to determine how many kinds of activity level exist, and how these might differ from each other both qualitatively and quantitatively.

In sum, research is needed that focuses on the issue of definition, standardization, and the multidimensionality of activity level/hyperactivity under the broad rubric of construct validity. The results of such studies would allow for the advance of theory and the development of adequate measurement devices, or the reconsideration of existing theory and modifications of currently employed devices. Although the intuitive approach is at times seen as adequate, it is the resulting lack of generalizability and control that severely limits the utility of previous efforts. Assessment cannot be considered to be independent of the etiology and theoretical basis of hyperactivity.

Review of Existing Scales

Child Rating Scale

Purpose and format: The *Child Rating Scale* (CRS) was developed by McConnell and his colleagues as a concurrent measure of activity level, to be used along with the ballistograph, a mechanical measure of activity level. The ten items on the CRS are rated by the user on a four-point continuum from "no, never" to "yes, all the time." The source of the items is not specified, although the authors state that "the scale attempted to include descriptive terms most often used in describing the syndrome of hyper-kinesis, with an emphasis on those characteristics related to actual body movement" (p. 648). The scale is completed by an observer. No directions for the training of raters are provided. Ratings are to be assigned based on the observer's impressions of the child over a three-day period.

Reliability: Test-retest over a one-week period on 57 moderately retarded subjects, ages six to 15 (ranging from hypoactive to hyperactive), was reported to be .86. Interrater reliability or internal consistency estimates are not reported.

Validity: The correlations with performance, measured using the ballistograph for the same 57 subjects, was .20.

Norms: None are provided, although males were rated as being more active than females.

Recommendation: The use of this scale is not recommended in its present form, due to the following reservations: (1) the high reliability coefficient could be attributed to variability in subjects' age and sex; (2) failure to give directions for training raters and not providing interrater reliabilities speaks against its utility; (3) the low correlation with the ballistograph raises questions about the validity of the instrument; (4) normative data are absent (what score should be considered hyperactive, etc.); (5) subjects on whom data are reported, constitute an extreme group, not readily generalizable to other populations; and (6) at least six single items ask two questions. In this regard, the structure of items appears poor and could present problems to users.

Classroom Behavior Inventory

Purpose and format: The *Classroom Behavior Inventory* (CBI) is a comprehensive instrument that provides assessments of school-age children on social, emotional, and task-oriented dimensions. Ratings of each child's behavior are completed by the classroom teacher. A variety of forms have been devised that allow assessments from preschool through the 12th grade. Depending upon the form used, and the grade level of the child, as many as 17 simple and 3 complex dimensions of behavior are assessed.

Items were developed based on the expertise of the authors, teachers' suggestions, and research findings on classroom behavior. Five items combine to produce a hyperactivity score for the child being rated. All items are rated using a four-point scale ranging from "not at all like" to "very much like." This subscale is present across all forms of the CBI.

Reliability: Reliability data in the form of internal consistency, stability, and interrater reliability estimates are presented for selected scales only. Overall, internal consistency estimates for the different scales appear high. The only reported indices for the hyperactivity scale are restricted to a sample of 7th graders, on whom ratings were obtained, indicating an internal consistency estimate of .93. While not given for the hyperactivity scale, the remaining scales on the inventory tend to have both low to moderate test-retest (over four months) and interrater reliabilities. Comprehensive reliability data across all scales are incomplete.

Validity: The CBI was developed using factor analytic methods, with no independent investigations directed towards establishing validity. Schaefer et al. suggest the existence of construct validity, yet evidence is not presented to support claims for the validity of the scale as a primary measure of hyperactivity.

Norms: No norms are provided nor are means, variances, and/or standard errors presented for the hyperactivity scale.

Recommendation: As a screening/selection device, the hyperactivity subscale is not recommended. Data are incomplete and scattered; small samples abound, with no definition of what types of children constitute the reference groups. The CBI appears to be an evolving research device, on which more work is needed. Also, the few items on the hyperactivity subscale (five) make the assessment process somewhat precarious.

Classroom Observation Code (COC)

Purpose and format: This recently developed instrument, is an observation system used in the classroom by trained observers in order to identify hyperactive children. Ratings are made on 14 categories that describe the child's behavior. Approximately 20 minutes of observation time is required to complete the rating for a child. To date, the authors suggest use with children ages 6 to 12 in classrooms characterized as "traditional."

Reliability: After 50 hours of training, five out of eight trainees were judged qualified as raters. The standard for interrater agreement was 70 percent accuracy of ratings. Examining the consistency of ratings by raters within the 14 categories, revealed a range of 33 to 96 percent agreement when there was behavior to be observed, with a mean agreement level across categories of 73 percent. Ratings over time revealed no significant shifts in assessments.

Validity: Five out of the 14 rated categories were found to be capable of discriminating hyperactive from nonhyperactive children. However, while statistically significant as discriminators, a high rate of false negatives (hyperactives) and false positives nonhyperactives) were noted, averaging approximately 25 percent for each group.

Norms: No norms are available.

Recommendation: This observational system has potential, and continued research should lead to significant modifications, such as the deletion of factors that account for small amounts of variance. It could readily be employed ,in context with other instruments, to assist in identification decisions, a sound and too infrequently used strategy. As a classroom observation schedule, the use of the COC may be prohibitive. The amount of training necessary, and marginal rates of inter-observer agreement make its utility questionable and possibly cost-inefficient.

Hyperactivity Rating Scale

Purpose and format: The *Hyperactivity Rating Scale* (HRS) is the result of reformulation, restructuring, and reanalyses of the original *Classroom Behavior Inventory* (Schaefer et al., 1966) discussed earlier in this chapter. Development of the HRS began by choosing 10 of the subscales from the CBI. Following considerable analyses, the scale is now represented by 11 factoral dimensions, each evaluated by three items. Items are completed by the classroom teacher, using a five-point rating scale from "never observed" to "always observed."

Selection of subscales to assess hyperactivity was based on the expert judgment of the authors. Factor analytic methods, using data gathered on a group of male kindergarten students (N = 320), from middle-class, predominantly Caucasion homes, have provided the basis for the final form of the HRS.

Reliability: No reliability information is reported.

Validity: The absence of reliability information is interesting, insofar as there is literature available relating to validity and norming efforts. The authors' early efforts at validity resulted in disappointingly low validity coefficients. This has been attributed to a tendency of teachers to generalize impulsive behaviors in children and label these hyperactive, and the low reliability of CBI scales, making screening with the HRS difficult.

More recent research on the earlier version of the HRS appears lacking, failing to provide clear evidence of the validity of this tool. The validity data reported, are based on factoring of response data obtained over a large sample of students in grades kindergarten through four. Independent studies (apart from the refactoring process) are not mentioned. By the authors' own admission, there appears to be considerable overlap between scores of hyperactive and nonhyperactive children, based on available data.

Norms: Norms based on 1,140 Caucasian children, rated by their teachers are available. While the model used by the authors to develop norms appears adequate, it may be premature. Issues still remain unresolved as to the validity and reliability of the HRS and, consequently, the utility of norms is questioned.

If one were to accept the scale as it stands, the norms described are good. Some concerns relate to the fact that the norms are available for whites only, and that no normative data for a "hyperactivity/activity level score" are given. The authors suggest, however, that five to nine of the HRS subscales go together to constitute a measure of hyperactivity.

Recommendation: Seemingly, the HRS has the potential to become a first-rate screening/assessment tool for identifying hyperactive children. At this stage, however, research is needed to insure users of its value. Reliability and independent validity studies are especially warranted. The specific matter of a score composite that can represent an index of hyperactivity/activity level needs to be addressed and discussed. The scale in its present form would be useful to the researcher, but practitioners in the field should view it cautiously.

Rating Scales for Hyperactive and Withdrawn Children

Purpose and format: These scales were developed to assist in the early identification of hyperactive and withdrawn children in a preschool setting. Items on the scales were developed based on the expertise of the authors.

Ratings are completetd by the child's teacher. Six behavioral descriptors of hyperactives, and three additional ones for the withdrawn dimension are used on an 11-point continuum. For each descriptor, from three to six of the positions of the continuum are operationally defined to assist the rating.

Reliability: Data, in the form of interrater reliability, are presented. The discussion of these data indicates that for male subjects, reliability ranged from .75 to .94 for the six hyperactive items, and from .88 to .93 for the three withdrawn items. For females, reliabilities were quite homogeneous, averaging .94 on the hyperactivity items and .95 on the withdrawn items. Other indices (test-retest, internal consistency) of reliability are not reported.

Validity: Items were assigned to scale membership, based on factor analyses, and, thus, claims for validity are grounded in this empirical technique. The proportion of variance accounted for by the two factors of hyperactivity and withdrawal is not specified. For males, a single bipolar factor was found; hyperactivity, whereas for females two factors; hyperactivity and withdrawn, were observed. Manipulation of ratings, as suggested by the authors, is to compute scores on both dimensions for both males and females. Although analyzed separately, one set of weights is suggested for use with both males and females.

Norms: The authors provide normative interpretations based on factor scores. These are based on 202 subjects tested in the original development of the scale. Predominantly white children, sampled from a narrow geographic region, limit the adequacy of the norms. Identical treatment of males and females introduces additional error in the utility of the norms. No attempt is made at specifying critical levels of activity (e.g., at what point along the hypothetical continuum does activity level become hyperactive?).

Recommendation: The scale seriously lacks attention to the criteria of external validity, as well as comprehensive reliabiilty documentation. The effort at establishing norms is laudable, but incomplete. The scale should be used with caution. As a basic research device it deserves the attention of specialists to assist in its development. Its potential with older groups might also be considered.

The Schenectady Kindergarten Rating Scales (SKRS)

Purpose and format: The SKRS is a battery of teacher-administered behavior-rating scales, developed as a means of screening large numbers of kindergarten children who may experience difficulty in school, due to language, motor, cognitive, and/or developmental deficiencies. Thirteen scales—each being a single-item category—are rated by the teacher. Ratings may be attempted as soon as one week after the teacher has first had contact with the children. Identfiication of two types of hyperactive children is possible: (1) low-ability hyperkinetic (those obtaining deviant scores on the impulse control, ability, clarity of speech, and cooperation with adults scales), and (2) hyperkinetic (those receiving deviant scores on the impulse control, cooperation with adults, and "some" of the ability scales). Sources for items and the rationale for scale points are not clearly made, nor is a rationale presented to justify the composition of scales within the hyperkinetic dimensions.

Reliability: Interrater reliability is presented. Using two independent raters, the scales average approximately 85 percent agreement when one scale-point deviation is allowed. Test-retest reliability over five months is quite variable over the 13 scales, ranging from .55 to .74.

Validity: The authors cite face validity for the scales. Also, their discussion of the predictive validity of the scales appears to be more within the domain of concurrent validity, given the criterion of first-grade teacher ratings a year later. Sufficient validity data are not available. The frequency of misclassification on the hyperkinetic dimensions appears high.

Norms: Although norms are provided, their generalizability may be questioned, since only children from Schnectady were included in the study. The basis for deviant scores, which defines classification, is not empirically justified. To be considered deviant on a particular scale, a rating at or below that of 25 percent of the normed population must be assigned. The norm group, which is characterized as predominantly white and middle class, includes approximately 2,900 children compiled over three years. Of any scale developed to assess hyperactivity, this represents, by far, the most extensive attempt at developing a base for the development of norms.

Recommendation: The instrument has an elaborate and large data base. The primary problems would appear to be potentially biased norms, inadequate documentation of interrater reliability, no apparent basis for defining deviant scores, and validity data (concurrent vs. predictive) that are interpretable in a variety of ways. Two additional points deserve attention. First, while a theoretical basis for classification of hyperactives is not presented, those scales that do contribute to this classification appear to be narrowly conceived. Second, each scale is measured by one item, a broad descriptive category, and ratings are given on a five- or seven-point continuum. The scale's length might permit exceedingly high measurement errors. As a procedure for focusing teacher judgments, the scale would seem to hold promise. However, its use is recommended only as a secondary or back-up cross validating procedure to other methods and scales.

Teachers Rating Scale (TRS) (recently being labeled the Hyperkinesis Index—Teachers)

Parent Rating Scale (PRS) (recently being labeled the Hyperkinesis Index—Parents)

Purpose and format: The two *Conners Rating Scales* were developed from Eisenberg's early efforts at devising a scale for teachers. Each instrument is composed of five factors: conduct problem, inattentive-passive, tension-anxiety, hyperactivity, and sociability. Ten items on both the teacher and the parent questionnaires measure the hyperactivity subscale. Items are rated for the child by the parent or teacher using a four-point continuum, ranging from "not at all" to "very much." Both parent and teacher scales are now distributed by Abbott Laboratories, North Chicago, Illinois 60064. The subscales measuring hyperactivity are probably the most frequently used in both research efforts studying hyperactivity and in field settings where documentation of a child's activity level is desired. The source of items for the scales was drawn from teachers who had worked with hyperactive children.

Reliability: Test-retest reliability estimates for the teacher questionnaire over a one-month period have been reported for the five subscales, and range from .72 to .91. The reliability for the hyperactivity scale is .84. Internal consistency indices are not available for subscales on either the parent or teacher questionnaires. Conners has reported the correlation between mother and father ratings of their children across the scales to average .85.

Validity: Many investigations have used the TRS and PRS on a pre-post basis, studying sensitivity of the scales to changes in behavior, as a result of drug treatment. These investigations have found that the scales are capable of noting scale score changes. Beyond these studies, validity information tends to be restricted to empirical validity claims, based on the factor analytic methodology used to define the scale's dimensions. A replication of Conners' analysis has recently been completed confirming, in part, Conners' original findings (Werry et al., 1975). The greatest exception to this comparison, were instances where the hyperactivity subscale joined with the intensive-passive subscale. These authors are critical of validity claims based on the scale's ability to be sensitive to changes in scores following treatment. In this context, validity information is narrowly focused.

Norms: The TRS and PRS are two of the few instruments reporting attempts at norm development. These data clearly reveal large differences in the scores obtained between hyperactive and nonhyperactive children. However, data are presented only for the Teacher Rating Questionnaire. Data were established using 68 hyperactive children and 223 nonhyperactive children. Participants who were rated by teachers spanned grades kindergarten through six. When the researchers attempted to establish more comprehensive norms using subjects rated by teachers from New Zealand, (N = 418), Champaign, Illinois (N = 291), and from New York City (N = 92), they observed a statistically significant mean difference between the Champaign group and the combination of N.Y.C. and New Zealand students. This difference is potentially attributable to a variety of factors, beginning with the representativeness with which samples were drawn, and the lack of an absolute, rather than a relative notion of what activity level represents.

Recommendation: *The Conners Scales* are unquestionably the most commonly used instruments. While a significant data base is accumulating, it is far from being considered the standard against which other measures should be judged. Psychometric data are more readily available for the teacher scales than the parent forms, yet in both cases available information is piecemeal and spotty (e.g., reliability data). In addition, it is distressing to note the lack of data addressing the validity of the instruments. While efforts at the development of norms are continuing, current data should be considered, with caution given the other dimensions for norms that must be considered such as sex, social class, age, etc.; since the literature consistently reports differential activity level in children as related to these variables. These dimensions deserve attention in any effort at establishing norms. If we are to give serious consideration to these scales as usable indices, more attention must be given to conforming to standards of education/psychological tests as described in the APA/AERA/NCME standards manual.

Other investigators should be encouraged to assist in the documentation of the these scales, by contributing their data when available. Data obtained through the use of these measures should be considered valuable and their utility maximized when concurrent measures can be gathered to assist decision making.

Werry-Weiss-Peters Activity Scale

Purpose and format: This scale is unique, insofar as it is designed to assess the activity level of the child exclusively. The measure attempts to quantify activity level, by isolating specific environments where behavior may be observed. The 31 items on the scale are rated for each child on a three-point continuation of "no-some-much." The scale is completed by the child's parents and teacher in order to obtain an activity level score.

Reliability: No reliability information was reported.

Validity: Studies correlating ratings on the WWP and mechanical measures of activity level have reported low correlations. A factor-analytic investigation revealed that seven stable and independent dimensions exist.

Norms: No norms are available.

Recommendation: Although the use of this scale has declined, the focus and specificity of the measure warrant further investigation. Use of the scale as a selection/identification tool by itself is not recommended, but as a screening instrument it may hold promise.

Conclusions

Based on the review of the instruments in the first section of this chapter, a number of conclusions can be drawn:

1. *A variety of behavioral assessment scales and techniques to assess activity level have been devised.* Obviously, there is a high degree of interest in this topic. Activity level, and specifically hyperactivity, is a variable of "high visibility" and great concern as it effects the developing child. It is noteworthy that when studies have attempted to intercorrelate ratings obtained across many of these measures, correlations have tended to be moderate (r's of .5 to .7). Although there is undoubtedly some shared variance across these instruments, further work at defining the nature of the construct seems most appropriate.

2. *The majority of instruments have documented interrater reliability and, while not always high, they tend to be acceptable.* This conclusion is a good sign, but it also points to a potential problem inherent in some of the measures. The positive side reveals that, since measures are characteristically completed by a second party (parent, teacher, physician, etc.), the behavioral attributes being considered are concrete and stable enough to permit accurate appraisal by a variety of raters. The negative aspect may be that scales are too narrowly conceived, with the result that perhaps systematic, although transitional behaviors, are being overlooked. In effect,

what is rated is adequate, but perhaps not enough is being evaluated by any one measure.

3. *Other evidence that relates to aspects of reliability is typically lacking, e.g., test-retest, internal consistency, standard errors of measurement.* This is a serious shortcoming. Users are left to their own best guesses as to the scale's reliability and, thus, in any investigation are compelled to compute their own estimate. The problem is that users are not informed of the accuracy and consistency of the scores being obtained. Given the level of statistical sophistication exhibited by the majority of developers in the preparation of their scales, it is almost embarrassing to find that estimates of reliability are not reported.

4. *Authors often make no attempt at improving the reliability of their measures.* A variety of techniques exist to improve the reliability of a scale. This is most typically achieved by increasing the number of items used to measure the behavior in question. The measurement methodologies used by authors are well suited to providing information as to which items to delete and to which cluster items belong. Yet, researchers have not gone back to add items to scales. Thus, a great many measures employ from five to 10 items, where parallel/equivalent items might have been added to the measure, in order to improve the reliability of scale scores obtained.

5. *Independent validity studies are seriously lacking.* When factor-analytic procedures are used in the development of a scale, the procedure becomes an end in itself and, somehow, one is to believe, guarantees validity. Factor analyses are good at identifying the dimensionality of a subset of items and when item responses are weighted by factor loadings, the resulting scores are maximally internally consistent. However, this is not proof of validity in and of itself. What is needed are studies specifically designed to assess the validity of these measures. Also, cross-validation efforts should be considered and implemented.

6. *The source of items on scales often lack any theoretical rationale.* Most scales derive their items from the expert opinion of the authors. This may yield a measure that too strongly represents the author's biases and fails to tap behaviors also characteristic and important in identifying the behavior under scrutiny; the result can be a scale that is narrowly focused. This may explain why items on scales appear to center in one specific location, e.g., in school, with peers, on task, etc.

7. *Few attempts to establish norms are found.* Empirical standards by which activity level is evaluated simply do not exist. Attempts to build norms for a few instruments appear to have serious shortcomings. In most cases, the user must arbitrarily define the critical cutoff. The danger in such

TABLE 1

Summary of Instruments

Title	Classroom Behavior Inventory	Child Rating Scale	Werry-Weiss-Peters Activity Scale	Classroom Observation Code	Teacher/Parent Rating Scales	Rating Scale for Hyperactive and Withdrawn Children	Schnectady Kindergarten Rating Scales
Author(s)	Schaefer et al., 1966	McConnell et al., 1968	Werry et al., 1968	Abikoff et al., 1974	Conners, 1969	Bell et al., 1972	Conrad and Tobiessen, 1969
Focus	Social, emotional, and task-oriented school behaviors	Activity level	Activity level	Hyperactivity	Behavior problems, attention, anxiety, activity level and sociability	Hyperactivity and withdrawing	Language, gross motor and cognitive development
Format	4-point rating scale	4-point rating scale	3-point rating scale	Rating scale	4-point continuum	11-point continuum	Rating scale
Reliability*	.93/NR	NR/.86	NR/NR	NR/NR	NR/.84	NR/NR	NR/.55 to .74
Validity†	NR	$r = 20$ with ballistograph	Low correlations with mechanical measures	5 or 14 rated categories discriminated hyperactive from non-hyperactive	Pre-test/post-test change	Factor analysis	Face validity
Norms	NR	NR	NR	NR	391 children	202 children from original population	2900 children
Primary user	Teacher	Observer	Observer	Researcher	Teacher/parent	Teacher/parents	Teacher

NR = Not reported or insufficient information
* Internal consistency test-retest
† Attempts at establishing validity

practices is clear. Just as there is a dire need for validity investigations, there is a commensurate need for norming investigations.

From the evidence presented here, no single measure can be recommended for use in screening large groups of children with a resultant high degree of confidence in the identification/selection data. This problem (or state of affairs) does not exist because the assessment of activity level is complex and fraught with pitfalls. Rather, it is a result of piecemeal, one-shot inquiries, designed without regard for follow-up studies and improvement. What is lacking are carefully controlled, long-term investigations that will result in the availability of respectable measures of activity level. The review in the second part of this chapter points to efforts in this direction. Although much needs to be done to improve the assessment of activity level, much of the information that has been reviewed here illustrates that attempts are being made. For the practitioner, as well as the researcher, many of these instruments can provide a starting point for further research in the areas of hyperactivity and activity level.

References

ABIKOFF, H., GITTELMAN-KLEIN, R., and KLEIN, D. F. *Validation of a Classroom Observation Code for Hyperactive Children.* Unpublished manuscript, Long Island Jewish-Hillside Medical Center, Glen Oaks, N.Y., 1976. (NIMH Grant #MH18569).

ARNOLD, L. E. and SMELTZER, D. J. Behavior check-list factor analysis for children and adolescents. *Arch. Gen. Psychiat.* 1974, 30:799-804.

BANHAM, K. M. *Activity Level Rating in a Testing Situation for Infants Two Months to Two Years.* Unpublished manuscript, 1967.

BELL, R. O. Adoption of small wrist watches for mechanical recording of activity in infants and children. *J. Except. Child Psychol.* 1968, 6:302-305.

BELL, R. Q., WALDROP, M. F., and WELLER, G. M. A rating system for the assessment of hyperactive and withdrawn children in preschool samples. *Amer. J. Orthopsychiat.* 1972, 42(1):23-24.

BLUNDEN, D., SPRING, C., and GREENBERG, L. M. Validation of the classroom behavior inventory. *J. Consulting and Clin. Psychol.* 1974, 42(1):84-88.

CHESS, S. Diagnosis and treatment of the hyperactive child. *N.Y.S. J. Med.* 1959, 60:2379-2385.

CONNERS, C. K. A teacher rating scale for use in drug studies with children. *Amer. J. Psychiat.* 1969, 126:884-888.

CONNERS, C. K. Pharmacotherapy of psychopathology in children. In Quay, H. C. and Werry, J. S. (eds.), *Psychopathological Disorders of Childhood.* New York: Wiley, 1972.

CONNERS, C. K. Rating scales for use in drug studies with children. *Psychopharmacol. Bull.* (Special Issues—Pharmacotherapy with children), 1973, 24-84.

CONRAD, W. G. and DUSELL, J. Anticipating the response to amphetamine therapy in the treatment of hyperactive children. *Pediatrics*. 1967, 40:96-98.

CONRAD, W. G. and TOBIESSEN, J. The development of kindergarten behavior rating scales for the prediction of learning and behavior disorders. *Psychol. in the Schools*. 1967, 4:359-363.

CROMWELL, R. L., BAUMEISTER, A., and HAWKINS, W. F. Research in activity level. In Ellis, N. R. (ed.), *Handbook of Mental Deficiency*. New York: McGraw, 1963, 632-663.

DAVIDS, A. An objective instrument for assessing hyperkinesis in children. *J. Learning Dis*. 1971, 4(9):499-501.

DELONG, A. What have we learned from psychoactive drug research on hyperactives? *Amer. J. Dis. Child*. 1972, 123:177-180.

DIELMAN, T., CARRELL, R., and LEPPER, C. Dimensions of problem behavior in the early grades. *J. Consulting Clin. Psychol*. 1971, 37(2):243-249.

EISENBERG, L. The management of the hyperkinetic child. *Dev. Med. and Child Neurol*. 1966, 8:593-598.

GITTELMAN-KLEIN, R., KLEIN, D. F., ABIKOFF, H., KATZ, S., GLOISTEN, A. C., and KATES, W. Relative efficacy of methylphenidate and behavior modification in hyperkinetic children: An interim report. *J. Abnorm. Child Psychol*. 1977 (in press).

GREENBERG, L. M., DEEM, M. A., and McMAHON, S. Effects of dextroamphetamine, chlorpromazine, and hydroxyzine on behavior and performance in hyperactive children. *Amer. J. Psychiat*. 1972, 129(5):532-539.

HUESSY, H. R. and COHEN, A. H. Hyperkinetic behaviors and learning disabilities followed over seven years. *Pediatrics*. 1976, 57(1):4-10.

KEOGH, B. Hyperactivity and learning disorders: Review and speculation. *Except. Child*. October, 1971, 101-109.

KNOBEL, M., WOLMAN, M., and MASON, E. Hyperkinesis and organicity in children. *Arch. Gen. Psychiat*. 1959, 1:310-321.

LAMBERT, N. M. et al. The hyperactivity-learning-behavior disorders project, 1976. University of California, Berkeley, School of Education.

LOO, C. and WENAR, C. Activity level and motor inhibition: Their relationship to intelligence test performance in normal children. *Child Dev*. 1971, 42:967-971.

McCONNELL, T. C. and CROMWELL, R. L. Studies in activity level: VII effects of amphetamine drug administration on the activity level of retarded children. *Amer. J. Ment. Deficiency* March, 1964, 68.

McCONNELL, T. R., CROMWELL, R. L., BIALER, I., and SON, C. D. Studies in activity level: VII. Effects of amphetamine drug administration on the activity level of retarded children. *Amer. J. Ment. Deficiency*. 1964, 68(5):647-651.

MORGAN, C. T. and STELLAR, E. *Physiological Psychology*. New York: McGraw-Hill, 1950.

POGGIO, J. P. and SALKIND, N. J. The development of a behavioral assessment battery to assess hyperactivity in children, 1977. The University of Kansas, School of Education.

POPE, L. and POPE, M. Measurement of motor activity in human subjects. *Percept. and Motor Skills*. 1969, 29:315-319.

RAPOPORT, J. and BENOLT, M. The relation of direct home observations to clinical evaluations of hyperactive school age boys. *J. Child Psychol. and Psychiat.* 1975, 16:141-147.

REED, J. D. Spontaneous activity of animals: A review of the literature since 1929. *Psychol. Bull.* 1947, 44:393-412.

ROSS, D., and ROSS, S. *Hyperactivity: Research, Theory, Action.* New York: Wiley, 1976.

SALKIND, N. J. and POGGIO, J. P. The measurement of activity level in children. Paper presented at the annual meeting of the American Psychological Association, Chicago, Ill., 1975.

SALKIND, N. J. and POGGIO, J. P. The measurement of hyperactivity: Trends and issues. In Fine, M. J. (ed.), *Principles and Techniques of Intervention with Hyperactive Children.* Springfield, Ill.: Charles C Thomas, 1977.

SANDOUAL, J. The measurement of the hyperactive syndrome in children. *Review of Educa. Res.* 1977, 47:293-318.

SCHAEFER, E. S., DROPPLEMAN, L. F., and KALVERBOER, A. F. *Development of a Classroom Behavior Checklist and Factor Analysis of Children's School Behavior in the United States and the Netherlands.* Unpublished manuscript, Laboratory of Psychology, National Institute of Mental Health, 1966.

SCHAEFER, E. S. and ANRONSON, M. *Classroom Behavior Inventory.* Unpublished manuscript, National Institute of Mental Health, 1970.

SCHMITT, B. D. *The Hyperactive Child.* Paper read at the University of Kansas Medical Center, June, 1974.

SCHREGER, J., LINDY, J., HARRISON, S., McDERMOTT, J., and KILLINS, E. The hyperkinetic child: Some consensually validated behavior correlates. *Except. Child.* 1966, 32:635-637.

SCHULMAN, J. L., KASPAR, J. C., and THRONE, F. M. *Brain Damage and Behavior.* Springfield, Ill.: Charles C Thomas, 1965.

SIMPSON, D. D. and NELSON, A. E. Attention training through breathing control to modify hyperactivity. *J. Learning Dis.* 1974, 7:15-24.

SPRING, C., BLUNDEN, D., GREENBERG, L. M., and YELLIN, A. M. Validity and norms of a hyperactivity rating scale. *J. Special Educ.* 1977, 11(3):313-321.

STEWART, M., THACH, B. T., and FREIDIN, M. R. Accidental poisoning and the hyperactive child syndrome. *Dis. Nerv. Sys.* 1970, 31(6):403-407.

STEWART, M., MENDELSON, W., and JOHNSON, N. Hyperactive children as adolescents: How they describe themselves. *Child Psychiat. and Human Dev.* 1973, 4(1):3-11.

TOBIESSEN, J. and CONRAD, W. G. *The Schenectady Kindergarten Rating Scales, 1968 Standardization.* Unpublished manuscript, 1970.

TOBIESSEN, J., DUCKWORTH, D., and CONRAD, W. G. Relationships between the Schenectady Kindergarten Rating Scales and first-grade achievement and adjustment. *Psychol. in the Schools.* January, 1971, 8(1):26-36.

WERRY, J. Developmental hyperactivity. *Pediat. Clin. North Amer.* 1968, 15(3):581-599.

WERRY, J. Studies on the hyperactive child: IV An empirical analysis of the minimal brain dysfunction syndrome. *Arch. Gen. Psychiat.* 1968, 19:9-16.

WERRY, J. Diagnosis, etiology, and treatment of hyperactivity in children. *Learning Disorders, 3,* Special Child Publication, Washington, D.C., 1968.

WERRY, J. and QUAY, H. C. Observing the classroom behavior of the elementary school children. *Except. Child.* 1969, 35(2):461-470.
WERRY, J. and QUAY, H. The prevalence of behavior symptoms in young elementary school children. *Amer. J. Orthopsychiat.* 1971, 4(1):136-143.

CHAPTER 10

Diagnosis and Intervention: A Summing-Up

From the information available on hyperactivity, the accepted viewpoint here is that the term hyperactivity refers to a set of symptoms that reflect a variety of possible causes. The symptoms—inattentiveness, impulsivity, physical overactivity, excitability, and distractibility—are often present in early childhood, thereby giving credence to the concept of a developmentally based, constitutional hyperactivity. But, the symptoms may also appear after age four or five, thereby offering support for the view of a psychologically based hyper-reactivity. Some experts still believe that there is an organic basis to hyperactivity (i.e., brain damage, cerebral dysfunction, neurological impairment, etc.,); however, there is limited data, via neurological study, to support this position among the majority of children labelled hyperactive. More recently, diet factors have been presented as a possible cause of hyperactivity. The scientific literature, however, remains inconclusive as to the incidence and degree of food substance related hyperactivity. Diet, as with the other possible etiological factors, needs to be considered seriously, but may or may not be relevant with a given child.

While the condition tends to diminish in severity by adolescence, residuals persist (i.e., poor grades, and personal and social adjustment difficulties). Intervention, rather than a "let's wait until he outgrows it" attitude, seems merited. The most prevalent form of intervention is medication, typically methylphenidate hydrochloride (Ritalin) and dextroamphetamine sulphate

233

(Dexedrine). As discussed in chapter one, these stimulant medications can produce a seemingly paradoxical effect in calming down a child.

There are a number of problems associated with the use of medication, however, some of which have been overly dramatized by the press. Aside from the hysteria over "drugging" children, there are more basic issues: Medication is ineffective for many children; problems of school learning and social-relationship difficulties remain even after the behavior has been drug-managed; there is the desire from a humanistic perspective to assist the child in learning to manage his own behavior.

Apropos to drug intervention, the comprehensive involvement of a physician is often difficult to obtain. The physician is usually an expensive, office-based person who is likely to have limited, isolated contacts with the child. It would seem inefficient for school- or clinic-based personnel, who have greater contacts with the child and family, to become dependent upon the physician to orchestrate the treatment. Yet, because of the possibilities for a physical basis to hyperactivity, including diet factors, judgment should be exercised as to when a referral for medical consultation is in order.

The major intervention needs to take place in the setting where the behavior is occurring and to be implemented by the persons having a frequency of contact with the child; such as parents, teachers, or other school-based consultants. Intervention needs to be concerned with behavioral management, so the child and others can survive together; but, it also needs to focus on increasing the child's repertoire of positive, adaptive responses to his environment; and to facilitating the development of the child as a responsible, self-managing, and adequately learning individual.

From this viewpoint, there are several important considerations associated with diagnosis and treatment of hyperactivity.

1. Every hyperactive child is a unique individual. While there have been attempts to categorize subgroups of hyperactive children, generalization is tenuous, at best. The interactions of the child with persons in his environment will vary, often confounding simplistic cause-effect thinking. While one child is accepted by his parents as a highly active child, a similar child is viewed as a management problem. The interaction of the child with these psychologically important persons needs to be understood as a part of the diagnosis of hyperactivity and has key implications for planning the treatment.

2. As an adjunct to the first point, the normal variances of childhood need to be understood by the persons involved. Children do develop on different maturational time-tables and do not always do so evenly. These

thoughts underscore the importance of obtaining an extensive developmental history, including documenting the mother's condition during pregnancy, the circumstances of birth, post-natal events, and the subsequent developmental picture in all areas of functioning, against the background of the family context.

3. The recognition that there may be varied inputs to the child's behavior pattern argues for a comprehensive study of the child. The goal of the study is a differential diagnosis that looks at the child holistically. The study should include the earlier mentioned developmental history, as well as psychological assessment of cognitive, affective, and sensory-motor areas; psychoeducational assessment of the child's academic functioning; interviews with teacher and parents; direct observation of the child in different settings; and, most importantly, the child's perceptions of himself and others with regard to his hyperactivity. A medical consultation may be advisable to screen for neurological and diet-related factors. Such a referral is a matter of judgment based on the accumulated information.

4. Behavioral descriptions are likely to be more useful than diagnostic labels. The term "hyperactivity" itself, conjures up all sort of erroneous images in the minds of otherwise reasonable people: What is the child doing? How do others react? On what tasks does he do well or poorly? How do different levels and kinds of reinforcement affect the child? How does the child's behavior vary with the setting and demands?

These questions can be answered through informal and criterion-referenced assessment procedures and systematic task analysis. Standardized, norm-referenced tests can give useful information and classification data, but require the kind of supplementation as described, in order to produce the sought after differential diagnosis.

5. Multiple interventions may be appropriate. Many of the case studies presented in this book, exemplify the successful use of a particular approach. This is not meant to represent an argument for a unitary intervention, unless such a narrow intervention seems merited. From a research perspective, multiple interventions could be viewed as "sloppy" and not permitting a clear conclusion of success. From the viewpoint of the practitioner, however, helping the child to function appropriately, by whatever means are available, is usually a higher priority than scientific rigor.

Considering the "spread" of effects of the hyperactivity syndrome into school learning, socialization, and family areas, there are clearly several probable fronts on which intervention can simultaneously occur. For example, personal counseling may assist the child in achieving greater self-acceptance and in positive responsiveness to efforts at academic remediation. Perceptual-motor training might be focused on specific symptoms; while conjunctive biofeedback, or relaxation training could also be used to encourage the child toward greater self-management of his behavior. Diet management might serve to reduce some of the motor activity and concentration problems, but a behavior modification program may then be required to guide the child in acquiring more socially appropriate behaviors.

6. Intervention may need to occur in stages. This concept is different from the earlier descriptions of multiple interventions. In this case, certain changes may be worked on as prerequisite to subsequent interventions. An example would be a child whose behavior was so disordered and impulsive that behavioral management, through either drugs or an elaborate behavior modification program, was necessary, prior to involving the child in a sensory-motor or remedial academic program.

Family factors might be considered to be very important in the maintenance, if not the inception of the hyperactivity syndrome as well. The professionals involved will have to exercise judgment as to whether work with the family, concerning their perception of the hyperactive child and the role he plays in the family system, needs to occur before other interventions are initiated. The judgment could be to avoid intruding on the family system via counseling, but instead, to bring about change in the classroom via behavioral techniques, and then to move into greater family involvement.

7. Collaborative involvement can be extremely helpful. In the school setting, there are numerous persons who have significant contact with the hyperactive child. There are also persons whose expertise can contribute to the diagnostic and intervention programs for the child. In terms of classroom procedures, it makes sense for the teacher to be a main figure in terms of input and program development. But others ought to contribute also. The school psychologist, learning-disabilities teacher, resource-room teacher, and school social worker may all have something to offer by way of ideas or actual involvement.

The parents need to be actively included in the child's treatment. They know the child best, can share what has been attempted, and can contribute information about the child that could be very useful in program planning. Indeed, recent federal legislation (PL. 94-142) has mandated parent involvement in staffings and in the preparation of individual educational plans for children who require special services in order to maximize their educational opportunities.

When children are receiving medication, collaboration between the physician, home, and school is also vital. Typically, there is minimal to non-existent collaboration between the physician and school personnel, and yet, the monitoring of the effects of medication is highly recommended. While there may be a standard dosage, there are individual child tolerance levels, so that the effects of medication will vary from child to child. Usually, some regulation of dosage, or combination of medication is needed to achieve at the desired effect. There are even crucial questions associated with the desired effect. When the dosage effectively "subdues" the behavior, it may have a negative effect on learning capacity. Consequently, feedback on general classroom behavior, as well as how the child learns, should be valuable information for the physician.

It is likely, in many situations, that the school or parents will have to raise the question of systematic monitoring of the effects of medication. This is even more important if other educational, therapeutic, or management programs are being considered simultaneous to drug use. Behavior rating scales, daily or weekly report cards, or other forms of systematic monitoring of the child's behavior can be initiated by school personnel and the parents, in cooperation with the physician. Often, the lack of such monitoring is a function of the physician's busy schedule, or lack of experience with concerned school personnel.

It is the legitimate prerogative of parents and school personnel to initiate contact with the physician in order to discuss a monitoring system, if one has not been recommended. There is a sad history of children being placed on stimulant medication for extensive periods of time without monitoring, and with subsequent evidence that the medication failed to exhibit any therapeutic effect.

8. Home management problems often get ignored. The structure and demands of the public schools underscore the hyperactive child's problems with attention, impulsivity, and distractibility. School resources can be quickly mobilized to develop potentially helpful interventions in the school setting. What help is available, however, for the parents in relation to home management of the child?

Home and school can collaborate best when neither is slighted and both areas function supportively of each other. The same persons available to plan a school-based program can assist the parents in home-management procedures. Through consultation with school personnel, parents can (a) learn more about hyperactivity; (b) become aware of some options for managing the child at home; such as setting limits, using positive reinforcement, programing the child's time at home, "winding him down" for bed, and helping him deal with his own hurts and frustrations; (c) increase their awareness of how their needs and behavior interface with those of the child; and (d) receive appropriate support, understanding in their attempts to accept and cope with the child.

9. Measuring behavior before, during, and after, is an important way of judging what changes may have occurred in relation to a planned intervention. Parents and teachers usually do not need a systematic record of the child's problematic behavior in order to judge whether they feel that the child has a problem. But, with the teacher and parent becoming involved with the child, in attempts to modify the child's behavior, it is helpful to collect some data in order to objectify changes.

There are a number of rating scales that have been used by parents and teachers in establishing a base-line and assessing change. The preceding chapter discussed such scales and assumed a rather critical posture toward many of the instruments, based on their construction and established reliability and validity. In "real" situations, the selection of a rating scale will usually take into account the content validity of the items: Are the items rated in fact descriptions of the behaviors that people are concerned about? If so, the instrument will probably be useful in rating the frequency of those behaviors for purposes of assessing change, even if the instrument can be faulted psychometrically.

The direct measurement of behavior circumvents many of the psychometric issues about rating scales that concern people. The persons involved in programing with the child, can review their perceptions of problem behaviors. By operationalizing them, so that different persons can agree on what they feel the behavior is, procedures for observing the behaviors can be established. Convenience is an important factor. If the schedule or type of observation technique is too complex or demanding, given the available resources, people will either resist participation or become frustrated once they attempt to observe and record behavior.

An interesting phenomenon occurs when people get concerned with measuring behavior; they have to carefully think about what they want to measure. The decision to take measurements requires a clearer definition of the problem. The actual rating or measure moves the involved persons away from subjective impressions.

A problem associated with measurement is that too narrow a view of the problem may be assumed. If our definition is solely in terms of what we decide to measure, then we might ignore important aspects of the problem.

For example, "out-of-seat" or "on-task" behaviors are relatively easy to operationalize and measure. But, these behaviors say nothing of the child's self concept, peer relationships, or academic progress. The combination of systematic rating by teachers and parents, along with some direct observation of important behaviors in different settings, and formal and informal assessment of academic areas, would seem to constitute a more comprehensive approach to objectively measuring the child's hyperactivity and related problem areas.

10. Maintaining energy and motivation in coping with the child's behavior, and keeping frustration in check, can be challenging for any of the involved persons. Mutual support, regular communication, and a readiness to go back to the "drawing board" in order to rethink a strategy, are necessary ingredients on the part of the people involved in the intervention program. This is an especially important message for consultants who work with the teacher or parents initially in developing an intervention program, but who later break contact with these persons. The teacher or parents may feel very isolated and eventually become less willing to invest energy in the program.

The intervention strategy devised was in the final analysis, a hypothesis as to what might work. It is reasonable to expect that modifications in the program will be necessary, based on changes in the child's behavior and the judgment of the involved persons as to what might be more effective. Termination of the program will also become a concern if success is achieved. Questions regarding when and how to terminate the program (an abrupt stop of treatment, as opposed to a gradual fading-out procedure) will need to be considered. Perhaps at some point of reasonable success, the focus of the program will need to shift. These questions are usually best handled in a staffing situation and, especially where data, as well as opinion, is being shared.

Index